Other books of interest from Blackwell Scientific Publications

Professional Discipline in Nursing, Midwifery and Health Visiting
Second edition
R.H. Pyne
0 632 02975 7

The Research Process in Nursing
Second edition
Edited by D.F.S. Cormack
0 632 02891 2

Health Visiting
Second edition
Edited by Karen Luker and Jean Orr
0 632 03324 X

The Royal Marsden Hospital Manual of Clinical Nursing Procedures
Edited by A. Phylip Pritchard and Jane Mallett
Third edition
0 632 03387 8

The Royal Marsden Hospital Manual of Standards of Care
Edited by Joanna M. Luthert and Lorraine Robinson
0 632 03386 X

Journals of interest published by Blackwell Scientific Publications

Child: Care Health and Development
European Journal of Cancer Care
Health and Social Care in the Community
Journal of Advanced Nursing
Journal of Clinical Nursing
Journal of Nursing Management

Welcome Back to Nursing

Wendy Green

OXFORD

BLACKWELL SCIENTIFIC PUBLICATIONS

LONDON EDINBURGH BOSTON

MELBOURNE PARIS BERLIN VIENNA

© Wendy Green 1993

Blackwell Scientific Publications
Editorial Offices:
Osney Mead, Oxford OX2 0EL
25 John Street, London WC1N 2BL
23 Ainslie Place, Edinburgh EH3 6AJ
238 Main Street, Cambridge,
  Massachusetts 02142, USA
54 University Street, Carlton,
  Victoria 3053, Australia

Other Editorial Offices:
Librairie Arnette SA
2, rue Casimir-Delavigne
75006 Paris
France

Blackwell Wissenschafts-Verlag
Meinekestrasse 4
D-1000 Berlin 15
Germany

Blackwell MZV
Feldgasse 13
A-1238 Wien
Austria

First published 1993

Set by Best-set Typesetter Ltd.,
  Hong Kong
Printed and bound in Great Britain by
  Hartnolls Ltd, Bodmin, Cornwall

DISTRIBUTORS

Marston Book Services Ltd
PO Box 87
Oxford OX2 0DT
(*Orders*: Tel: 0865 791155
        Fax: 0865 791927
        Telex: 837515)

USA
Blackwell Scientific
Publications, Inc.
238 Main Street
Cambridge, MA 02142
(*Orders*: Tel: 800 759-6102
           617 876-7000)

Canada
Times Mirror Professional
Publishing, Ltd
130 Flaska Drive
Markham, Ontario L6G 1B8
(*Orders*: Tel: 800 268-4178
           416 470-6739)

Australia
Blackwell Scientific
Publications Pty Ltd
54 University Street
Carlton, Victoria 3053
(*Orders*: Tel: 03 347-5552)

British Library
Cataloguing in Publication Data

A catalogue record for this book is
available from the British Library

ISBN 0-632-03556-0

Library of Congress
Cataloging in Publication Data

Green, Wendy H.
    Welcome back to nursing /
Wendy Green.
    Includes bibliographical references
and index.
    ISBN 0-632-03556-0
    1. Nursing – Study and teaching
(Continuing education) – Great
Britain.   2. Employment re-entry –
Great Britain.   3. Nursing –
Vocational guidance – Great
Britain.   I. Title.
    [DNLM: 1. Employment.
2. Nursing.   WY 16 G798w]
RT76.G74   1993
610.73′069 – dc20
DNLM/DLC
for Library of Congress   92-49296
                                      CIP

Contents

Foreword   vii
Preface   ix
Acknowledgements   x

Part 1 – How It Was   **1**
1 Reminiscences   3
2 The Interim Years   17

Part 2 – Time to Return   **31**
3 Why Return?   33
4 What Does Retraining Involve?   42

Part 3 – Back to Practice   **53**
5 Has Nursing Changed?   55
6 Professional Practice, Knowledge and Skills   66
7 Practical Experience   79

Part 4 – Forward to the Future   **91**
8 Do I Still Want to Return?   93
9 Training and Professional Development   109
10 The Future   122

Index   132

Foreword

I was extremely pleased to be invited to write the foreword to this book. Nursing is passing through a period of major change, both in terms of education and practice. It holds innumerable challenges for those who continue to practice. For those who have had a break in practice, for whatever reason, the changes must seem almost insurmountable. The comfort is, of course, that the essence remains unchanged – the objective of all our endeavours being to give empathetic, safe, loving and effective care to our patients and clients.

Those who are considering returning to nursing will find much to reassure and help them in the text. It does not attempt to hide the challenges but uses a mixture of pragmatism, good humour and common sense which sets the major changes into context and shows how nurses and nursing continue to contribute in a substantial way to the delivery of health care in the United Kingdom.

Although written primarily for nurses, it will also have relevance for those considering returning to midwifery or health visiting.

In the course of my role as a senior member of staff of the statutory body which regulates nursing, midwifery and health visiting, I am in regular contact with large numbers of the 635,000 practitioners who are registered with the UKCC. One of the prime concerns amongst many of these practitioners is how to keep their knowledge base and professional practice up-to-date. This is a particular challenge for those who are returning to practice after a break. Not only is it necessary to brush the cobwebs off previous knowledge and skill, but also to subject that knowledge and skill to scrutiny under a fairly merciless spotlight, to ensure that it is accurate, relevant and sufficient. It is, of course, essential to learn how to complement such a process by recognizing the wide range of new skills, experiences and knowledge that have been acquired since last practising as a nurse. Life experiences are invaluable in our understanding of the needs of our patients and clients and their value should never be negated or diminished.

The wealth of anecdote in this book is particularly valuable in allowing the reader the opportunity of saying, 'that's how it was with me'. However, gently but firmly the text moves from what was, to what is now to be expected. For those considering returning to nursing this book will be invaluable.

For all the changes, we must never forget our prime function:

'The unique function of the nurse is to assist the individual, sick or well, in the performance of those activities contributing to health or its recovery (or to peaceful death) that he would perform unaided had he the necessary strength, will or knowledge. And to do this in such a way as to help him gain independence as rapidly as possible.'

Virginia Henderson
(The Nursing Process, edited by Charlotte R Kratz)

Welcome back to the family!

Margaret Wallace
Assistant Registrar
Educational Policy and Registration
UKCC

Preface

Return to Practise, recommendation 6 of the UKCC PREPP document will become a statutory requirement. This states that:

'When registered practitioners wish to return to practise after a break of five years or more, they will have to complete a return to practise programme . . .

All registered practitioners are accountable, but those doing a return to practise programme, despite having a registered qualification, would not be eligible to practise without supervision until the programme has been completed with a successful assessment of their professional competence.

On satisfactory completion of the return to practise programme, the individual will submit to the Council both evidence of completion and notification of practice. Return to practise programmes must meet the Council's requirements and be approved by a National Board. They will cover practitioners intending to work in the public and independent sectors.'

This book is a user-friendly account of the experiences of nurses who have taken the first steps in the process of returning to nursing. The initial misgivings and doubts about the ability to practise again are discussed. Their need for new knowledge and development of practical skills are explored together with the changes they have observed, including both the positive and negative ones.

Because the book is firmly based around the actual accounts of returning nurses over a number of years, there is an authentic ring to the topics included and the way in which they are covered. It is anticipated that this will allay fears and excite interest in picking up the threads of a career again.

It is not however an attempt to write an academic treatise about returning to work. To this end sub-headings and direct references are seldom used in the text. At the end of each chapter a list of books and articles are included which were both an inspiration and gave information for the chapter.

Whilst the book is primarily written around nursing, there are elements that may be of interest to those contemplating returning to midwifery or health visiting.

Wendy Green
June 1992

Acknowledgements

By its very style this book could not have been written without the valuable contribution from many nurses. In particular the hundreds of returning nurses who generously gave me permission to quote freely from them. The colleagues who read and commented on the early drafts and encouraged me to persevere are also to be thanked.

I am grateful to Tom Wise for interpreting my quotes into cartoons so aptly.

Above all my thanks go to Joy Carter for patience and promptness in producing the many copies of the manuscript.

Finally a thank you to my husband Len Green who was deprived of his Sunday walks whilst I was engaged in writing.

Part 1
How It Was

Chapter 1
Reminiscences

Ask any group of nurses what it was like when they trained and you will be immediately regaled with a variety of anecdotes. There is a school of thought in caring for the elderly that reminiscent therapy enables them to relate more effectively to the present. Some theorists however suggest that this can be dangerous if the links or connections are not made at the time, thus allowing reminiscing to descend into maudlin sentimentality or 'anecdotage', a term coined by some historians.

Whenever nurses are asked about their past nursing experiences most tend to see them through rose-coloured spectacles; time does tend to erode reality. They remember the grateful, undemanding patient and the tokens of their thanks but tend to forget the complaining unresponsive patient who often inconsiderately died. They remember the funny incidents and the games they played with other members of staff but tend to forget the sheer hard slog, the dirty, dangerous and unrewarding work that was part of nursing. They saw doctors as somewhere near God whose every command they obeyed, and failed to question the subservient role they played or the orders they were given.

It is useful however to see where we have come from and understand why it was like that, in order to make sense of and appreciate where we are going.

Dominance of matron

For many older nurses who trained in the 1950s and 1960s, some of whom are still nursing today, many in senior positions, Matron was the key person in the organization. She was the person to be respected, feared and obeyed, yet never to be forgotten; even today many nurses can recall her name often with a measure of affection. If you ask today's student nurses who their Director of Nursing Services is and if they have ever seen them, they will often be puzzled as to why you have even asked, and often will answer negatively.

In the early days of the NHS, Matron appeared to be totally in-

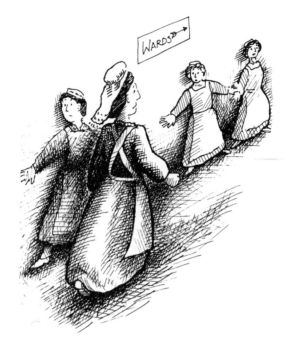

Matron in full flight.

destructable and unchallengeable. Looking back she (it was almost always 'she') was larger than life, a tall, well-proportioned woman whose appearance was enhanced by her striking uniform. An elaborately decorative starched cap covered severely restrained hair. This topped a dark, long-sleeved dress, which was sometimes covered by a crisp, white apron and usually trimmed with starched white collar and cuffs. The outfit was completed with thick, dark, Lisle or silk stockings and black low-heeled well-polished shoes.

Hattie Jacques captured this stereotyped picture admirably in the comedy films of the Richard Gordon 'Doctor' books, and in the *Carry On* films which had a 'medical' theme. What poor student nurse or even young doctor could fail to be intimidated by this 'dragon' as she almost literally sailed down the hospital corridors and through the wards, reducing all she met to shivering wrecks. As one nurse recalls:

'Matron's visit put you on edge, she was so starchy and critical. She visited the ward every morning and the work was organized around this visit. Bed wheels had all to be turned in, sheets and bed cover corners were folded with military precision, patient comfort was not considered. Lockers and bed tables were cleaned and only five items per patient were allowed on top. Matron greeted every patient, many of whom she knew by name, with the sister or senior nurse introducing those patients Matron had not met. Most of the nurses on the ward made themselves scarce during the visit but if by chance you inadvertently strayed across her path you could expect to be examined from head to toe. Any ladder or hole in your stockings, or spot or blemish on your starched white apron would be pounced upon and earn you a severe reprimand and dismissal to your room to repair the damage.'

Another nurse remembers an occasion when she was running down the long hospital corridor in order to catch a train home, having as usual come off duty late. She was stopped dead in her tracks by the stentorian boom of Matron's voice echoing down the corridor enquiring *'Fire, flood or haemorrhage, nurse?'*. By the time she stopped to give her lame excuse she had of course missed her train.

Strict discipline and obedience to the rules were instilled in nurses right from the outset of their training. One of the worst things that could happen to a student nurse was the summons to Matron's office at 9 AM. This was frequently given by the Home Sister at breakfast, making it impossible for the poor unfortunate to finish her meal. This was then followed by an agonizing wait in the outer office, under the sympathetic gaze of the secretary, which reduced even the toughest nurses to a state of panic as they frantically tried to think of an acceptable story to explain the sins of the previous day or night.

However, not all memories of Matron were negative, as shown by an obituary to Miss Smail, former Lady Superintendent of Nurses, printed in *The Pelican*, the Nurses League Journal of the Royal Infirmary of Edinburgh 1967:

> 'As we toured the wards she seemed to know all the patients and had a kindly word for the seriously ill. She had an intense love of, and pride in, her profession. She set high standards for herself and expected and obtained the same from her staff. She was a strict but sympathetic disciplinarian and had what one might call a "gentle firmness".'
>
> A.D. Stewart

Changes in management

Although the emergence of the 'matron' figure began only towards the end of the 19th century, her sphere of influence was already declining by the end of the Second World War. When the NHS was introduced in 1948, tripartite rule was established with doctors and administrators sharing the running of hospitals with the matron. The final blow came with the implementation of the Salmon reorganization in 1966 when the post of matron was abandoned. Nursing management was modernized with the introduction of nursing officers to achieve more efficient use of nursing staff.

It could be argued by some that Matron did not disappear but even today is a rose by another name i.e. Matron, Senior Nursing Officer, Director of Nursing Services. What has gone however is the supreme power and authority vested in one person to run the hospital. In today's world that would be neither possible nor desirable.

Bureaucratic organization

Synonymous with these memories of Matron was the control of nursing by the rules and regulations of the bureaucratic organization and its rigid hierarchy. Many of these controls were rooted in the desire to make nursing respectable, to tie it to the Victorian ideal of woman-hood, i.e. carefully supervised, closed institution, subordinate to men (doctors), underpaid with long hours and a short working life. This is well illustrated by the conditions of service for a student nurse entering training in 1960 at the Harrogate General Hospital (see Fig. 1.1). A male nurse who gave me this copy remembered how rigid hierarchy at the hospital prevented him as a student nurse from having meal or coffee breaks with his fiancée who was then a staff nurse. Later on the roles were reversed when he became a charge nurse and his wife, who was still a staff nurse, could not join him for meal breaks in the sister/charge nurse's dining room.

Many nurses will also remember how, as first year student nurses, they held the door open for second years' and above, and as second years' they held the doors for third years', and so on. They always stood when a senior nurse entered the room regardless of what they were doing at the time, and always addressed all staff by their surname with only senior staff having their name prefixed by a title.

Nurses were not expected to think for themselves or make decisions, this was the responsibility of someone more senior, as one nurse remembers:

'On handing over to the ward sister at the end of a very busy shift, she seemed more concerned that the stock bottles had not been counted rather than the fact that the patients had received care.'

A retired nurse who had recently received hospital care noted sadly:

'We worked hard and often thought we would give up, but our vocation kept us going. I'm sure some of the sisters who taught us would turn in their graves if they could come back and see how hospitals are run today.'

HARROGATE GENERAL HOSPITAL

Training allowances

1st Year £365 gross	Less £143 payable to the Hospital
2nd Year £390 gross	for board and residence, use and
3rd Year £420 gross	laundry of uniform.

All Student Nurses are required to be resident during the Introductory Course period, and are advised to be so during their first year.

On completion of her training the Student Nurse is given the opportunity, if suitable, to remain on the staff of the Hospital as a trained nurse and it is most desirable that she should make the most of this opportunity for at least 6 months.

As soon as she is a State Registered Nurse her salary commences at £690 per annum gross – special duty payments for Sunday and night duty.

Hours of duty

Day duty hours are arranged so that all nurses are on duty 42 hours between Sunday AM and Saturday PM. They are arranged the previous week by the Ward Sister as follows:

(1)   7.30 AM to 1.45 PM
(2)   2.30 PM to 9.30 PM
(3)   7.30 AM to 5.00 PM
(4)
(5)   Either 7.30 AM to 9.30 AM and 1 PM to 8.30 PM
(6)   or   7.30 AM to 1.15 PM and 5.00 PM to 8.30 PM
(7)   Day off.

Meal times are as follows and are not included in the hours of duty:

Breakfast	7.10 AM.
Coffee break	half an hour between 8.30 AM and 10.00 AM.
Dinner	half an hour at 12.30 PM or 1.15 PM.
Tea	half an hour between 4.00 PM and 5.30 PM.
Supper	half an hour at 7.00 PM or 7.30 PM.

Night Duty hours are arranged so that nurses work 34 hours during 9 consecutive nights, from 8.20 PM to 8.00 AM with 2 × 1 hour breaks for meals and rest. The remaining 5 nights in the fortnight are free of duty.

Annual leave

28 days per annum for 1st and 2nd year students, and 35 days per annum for 3rd year students.

Fig. 1.1 Harrogate General Hospital conditions of service in 1960. (Source: Harrogate Health Care.)

Nursing as a calling

Unfortunately most nurses, their employers and the general public remained rooted in this Nightingale ethic of caring as a duty, serving others subserviently. Nightingale commented 'They call it a profession but I say it is a calling'. For her it was tied up with a belief that she was performing a mission from God. The qualities of a 'good' nurse were: to be kind to patients, efficient, clean, neat and conscientious. As most nurses were recruited from the middle or working classes with relatively humble backgrounds, who needed to work for a living, they were willing to accept these conditions of work.

It is interesting to note that doctors declared on the one hand that book learning was of little value to nurses as all they had to do was carry out doctors' orders, yet at the same time *The Lancet* observed in relation to the debate on the need to change the conditions of nurses that all one needed to change was the restrictive discipline of the Victorian servant, i.e. compulsory attendance at meals, regulated bedtimes, system of late passes, fines for staying out late and the rigid hierarchy of social relations between staff.

The socialization of nurses, which imbued them with values and expectations designed to ensure they took their place in the system and thereby helped to keep it going on the same lines, served the bureaucratic system well. Examples of such diverse rules and regulations and infringements of personal liberty were:

- Beds made with meticulous hospital corners.
- Pillow case openings facing away from the door.
- All bed wheels turned inwards.
- Five items only allowed on a locker.
- Uniform not to be worn outside the hospital.
- Every nurse due on duty had to attend breakfast at 7 AM, or 7 PM when on night duty.
- Being told at breakfast that you were on night duty that night, then having to work until mid-day.
- Being woken for trivial reasons.
- Having unwanted pregnancy reported to the school staff.

And so on; this list is not exhaustive.

Administrative neatness and convenience were all important. One did not question the system, therefore change was inconceivable. There was a correct answer to all problems, but insecurity, lack of confidence and assertiveness, and unrealistic expectations of others led nurses to pretend to themselves and others that they knew it all and were capable of anything. In fact quite the reverse was true; training in the old days did little to make the trainee a strong independent person, able to make decisions based on knowledge and to be accountable for those decisions.

Some of the most striking features nurses note when they return to the clinical situation today is the warm, welcoming friendliness of all the staff in the team, with the use of christian names the most notable evidence of this; also the relaxed atmosphere on the ward with nurses actually sitting down and talking to patients; and finally the permission to say no and mean it and have this accepted without question or argument.

Training schools

Many nurses recall, with pride and a measure of affection, the name of their training hospital e.g. Jimmy's, Guy's, Tommy's, St Mary's, Addenbrooke's, the Bristol Royal Infirmary and so on. This abiding interest in their training hospital is perpetuated in the number of guilds or associations of nurses which still exist and whose members meet regularly to exchange news but more importantly to keep in touch with what is happening in their old hospital and in nursing in general.

Years ago, where you trained was felt to be important, especially when applying for posts in other hospitals. This might well stem from the fact that, although between 1919 and the establishment of the NHS in 1948, registered nurses might share a common certificate, their practical training and educational experience could vary widely. Individual hospitals were jealous of their reputation, both for their hospital examinations and state final examinations. This variation might well begin with selection for training.

In the immediate post-war years job opportunities for women were on the whole limited to teaching, nursing, secretarial and shop work. Nursing provided a great opportunity for women to leave home and live and work independently. Depending on the training school, nurses would not necessarily be selected on the basis of academic achievement. As mentioned earlier, such characteristics as honesty, obedience, conscientiousness and cleanliness were considered to be far more important.

Social conditions

Probationers were usually required to live in hospital accommodation. This might be a nurses' home in the hospital grounds, strictly supervised by Home Sister, or a nearby hostel which also had a resident warden. Sometimes you might be lucky and have a room to yourself but two or three people sharing a room was very common. Cooking in the home was not encouraged, although tea and toast was allowed on days off. Doors were usually locked by 10.30 PM; access later than that was by a system of late passes which required night sister unlocking the door. This she had to fit around running the hospital so it sometimes meant a long wait whilst she dealt with a crisis.

It was a fair system in that nurses were protected from unwelcome visitors, and for people engaged in such hard work as nursing 10.30 PM was a reasonable time to go to bed. Of course for the ingenious mind there were always ways of entering a locked establishment if the need arose.

This is in sharp contrast to student nurses' life today. Although accommodation might still be provided, they are not obliged to use it. If they do they will have their own pass key to the outer door, which is locked at all times. Provision is made for the nurse to cook meals in the home and there is no restriction on visitors. A home warden is there during the day but this is more to ensure smooth running of the home than for disciplinary purposes.

As with accommodation, food used to be provided by the establishment with money deducted from pay. It was usually of indifferent quality and local cafés and restaurants were well used to nurses requiring cheap and nourishing meals. Visits home also provided welcome supplements which were shared with fellow nurses.

Social life on the whole was fairly restricted due partly to the unsociable hours nurses worked but also to the lack of private transport. Local theatres were usually quite generous with their complimentary tickets, which were snapped up by nurses, especially for popular shows.

Training

As for training, most practical skills were learned 'alongside Nellie' – usually a more senior student. This led to a great variation in the quality and standards of competence achieved. Theoretical sessions varied according to the type of training offered. After the initial, preliminary training in school, nurses might be required to attend occasional lectures by medical staff when it suited them and to attend nursing lectures from tutors at set times. This could well be in off duty or holiday time but there was no excuse for non-attendance. One nurse recollects attending a surgeon's lecture on abdominal surgery:

'I had been working the previous night and the lecture was from 11 AM–12 noon. I was due on duty the following night but there was no reprieve. As the lecture progressed I fought hard to keep my eyes open but nature had its way and I slept peacefully through the proceedings. I was rudely awakened at the end of the lecture by the irate surgeon who took a great delight in reporting me to the horrified Sister Tutor. My punishment was to borrow somebody's notes to write up the lecture before I was finally allowed to go to bed. The system was changed soon after that, to study blocks in the School of Nursing.'

Training depended heavily on repetition and rote learning rather than reasoning and rationale, in order to pass the state examinations. Nurses were not encouraged to ask questions or criticize nursing practice. Theoretical knowledge was very closely related to medical knowledge, with a concentration on anatomy, physiology, body systems and disease processes. This knowledge was tested with a written examination at the end of three years.

Practical skills were usually assessed on the wards either by the ward staff, if they had time, or more recently by clinical teachers. Although to many this might seem a reasonable system of testing whether a nurse could be admitted to the register, it has to be said that many a 'good' nurse was sabotaged by equipment.

Perils of equipment

It would often assume a life and identity of its own and strike back when you least expected it, and often at the most inconvenient time, as recounted by a clinical teacher assessing a student nurse on her dressing technique:

> 'In washing down the trolley, prior to laying it up, she (the student), possibly because of nerves, was over generous with the soap solution. There were bubbles everywhere, on the floor, on the nurse, on me and floating in the air. It took us nearly an hour to clear up the mess.'

Another piece of equipment which tested the unwary was the humble bedpan. Years ago, before disposables with plastic shells, bedpans were meant to last. They were made of shiny aluminium which was cold and noisy and were a source of pain and pleasure, comfort and discomfort to both the patient and the nurse.

An oft repeated incident was the nurse creeping around in the dark at 5 AM with a metal trolley full of warmed metal bedpans and hitting an obstruction, such as a carelessly left slipper or item of furniture, and the whole content of the trolley cascading noisily to the floor. No patient could sleep through that!

The nurse made a quick exit to the comparative haven of the sluice. Here however more danger lurked in the form of the bedpan washer, a malevolent piece of equipment out to catch the unwary nurse. In theory one was supposed to empty the contents of the pan down the toilet, then slide the soiled pan into the drop-down door of the washer. One then closed the door, pulled down an arm to seal it, then pulled or pushed a lever to wash the pan. The trouble was, if the seal was not made properly the door flew open and the poor unfortunate on the outside received an unexpected early shower.

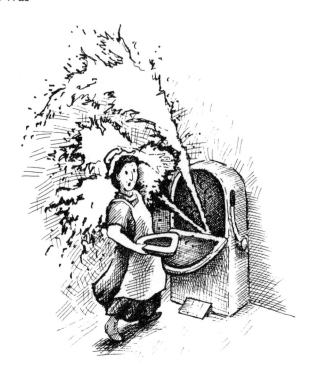

Going for an early shower.

Somehow bedpan mashers do not have the same character, although they can be brought to a standstill if a plastic shell is inadvertently added by an uninformed nurse.

When on duty nurses were never allowed to be idle. Many activities were undertaken which were not strictly nursing duties, such as damp dusting beds, lockers and bed tables, folding swabs and packing drums for autoclaving, and washing and rolling bandages. Polishing aluminium bedpans or washing down walls was often imposed as a punishment for disobedience.

Another source of trouble was the sterilizer in the treatment room; this was, of course, prior to the introduction of sterile supplies. The sterilizer was used to boil up a variety of objects, from instruments to bowls and receivers, rubber catheters and tubing, and even, on one occasion, all the ward's thermometers! It took several months for the unfortunate, enthusiastic nurse to pay for the replacements.

Before the days of a dipstick for testing for glucose in urine, a Bunsen burner was a standard piece of equipment in most sluices. This was used for other purposes than testing urine, as one nurse recounts:

'It was one of the jobs of the junior nurse to wash the masks and bandages, then boil them. They were usually put in a large aluminium bowl of water which was placed on a tripod over the Bunsen burner. Busy as usual, I set the masks and bandages over the Bunsen burner and went about my other duties. Suddenly an all pervading smell of burning filled my nostrils. The masks and bandages! I rushed to the sluice; too late – the water had boiled away leaving a brown and white mess in the bowl.'

Working in the operating theatres years ago could fill a nurse with fear and dread. Prior to the sterile supplies department, all instruments used in theatres had to be scrubbed clean by theatre staff then dried, polished and placed on shelves in glass-fronted cupboards in the correct order. Every instrument had a name and a correct place on one of the shelves; these all had to be learned by the theatre nurses.

Before surgery the instruments were packed into trays and boiled to sterilize them. There was a great deal of pride and satisfaction in seeing rows of gleaming intruments at the end of a busy operating day. However operating lists did not always run smoothly; some disasters remembered were:

- The time the unfortunate nurse leant against the light switch and plunged the theatre into darkness just as the operation was about to start.
- A surgeon almost scalding his hands when he plunged them into a freshly-made bowl of antiseptic solution which should have been cooled.

With all these activities going on how did the nurse find time for the patient? A justification for the patient-centred care advocated today is that under the task allocation system in which nurses worked years ago, patients did not get to know their nurses and nurses did not know their patients. This is always strongly contested by returning nurses who worked under that system.

Relationship with patients

What was very different in those days was that the patient stayed in hospital much longer, e.g. 14 days for a hernia repair, ten days for a normal birth and so on. The patients, of course, were not ill all that time and part of their rehabilitation was to help the nurses with some domestic chores, like taking round the teas and morning and evening drinks, putting flowers in vases and talking to other patients. Working alongside nurses like this meant that they had more personal contact with each other.

Another factor in the contact time was that nurses worked much longer hours than nurses do today; 50 hours was common 20 years ago, with much unofficial overtime being done as you were not allowed off-duty if your work was not completed. With only one and a half days off-duty, not always taken together, there was certainly much more opportunity for patients and nurses to get to know each other.

A third difference between then and now was the design of the ward. In the old, open, Nightingale type wards all the patients could see the nurses and could be seen by the nurses. Patients very quickly learned the nurses' names and developed preferences. They knew which nurse they could trust to boil their breakfast egg to their liking (and who would remember to write their name on their egg). They could identify the nurse who collected up all the false teeth to clean, then could not remember which teeth belonged to which patient. They knew who took the trouble to warm the bedpan before sitting the patient on it, and who responded promptly to a request for a pan or bottle.

Most patients appreciated the care they received and showed their appreciation in many small ways, like the sweet, fruit or cigarette slipped in the pocket for consumption later, and the saved newspaper or magazine for 'their' nurse to read in bed when finally off-duty.

Some patients and nurses formed even closer attachments, from friendship to proposals of marriage. Fortunately in the latter case most nurses realized these were made more out of gratitude than any personal attributes.

One nurse remembers with amusement the dashing RAF Officer who on discharge made arrangements to meet her and drive her to London to the Windmill Theatre where his uncle worked; needless to say she waited for him in vain. Another nurse promised she would marry a young man suffering from ulcerative colitis; later that night he died peacefully in her arms. On the neurology ward a nurse was proposed to by a wealthy young Arab Sheikh who developed a passion for her; sadly his brain tumour proved to be inoperable but he was sustained by his ardour.

Dealing with death

Most nurses remember patients they have cared for who were dying. A majority of the memories will be sad, occasionally tragic, but rarely funny. One nurse recounts sitting with a 40-year-old woman who was dying from cirrhosis of the liver. Near death the woman opened her eyes and looking straight at the nurse said, 'Is this it? Is my life over? It has hardly begun!' To a 20-year-old nurse this was very poignant.

Another nurse recalls the time she spent on an elderly care ward. One old lady who had not been a patient for long had her 90th birthday on the ward. The staff made a fuss of her, putting a ribbon in her snow-white hair, before she cut her birthday cake. She shed a few tears afterwards, and when the nurse asked why she said that this was the first birthday party she had had and the first cake made just for her. She died the next day.

Not all anecodotes were sad; even death could have its amusing side. A ward sister asked a fairly new student nurse to prepare the body of a patient, who had died and been laid out, for the relatives to view as they had arrived too late to see the man before he died. The student nurse busied herself behind the curtains.

When the relatives arrived the sister discreetly ushered them through the curtains, only to pull herself up in horror at the spectacle that greeted them. The body had been sat upright, glasses were perched on the man's nose and a newspaper had been placed between his hands. Fortunately the relatives did not see the man. Sister made an excuse to usher them out while she rectified the situation.

When the student nurse was asked for an explanation she said Sister had asked her to make the man look natural, so what was more natural than sitting up in bed reading a newspaper!

Young patients

Perhaps because they could relate personally to them, most nurses remember the young patients they cared for, particularly those whose condition was terminal or severely disabling. Like the promising young dancer who had to have his leg amputated. The night before surgery he was crying on the shoulder of the young nurse who was very sympathetic. This sympathy was soon shattered however by the staff nurse who was very religious and told the young man it was God's will and he must accept it. To the young nurse she said it was unprofessional to cry with patients; it looked weak, especially when he would need someone strong to rely on during the next few days.

As new motorways opened up across the country an increasing number of accident victims were admitted to neighbouring hospitals, young motor cyclists being particularly vulnerable to head injuries. One nurse in Staffordshire remembers one such victim, a 17-year-old boy with severe head injuries. He had burr holes to relieve the pressure and remained unconscious for many weeks. The nurse recalled with great satisfaction that she was there when he finally walked out of the ward, on his way to rehabilitation.

Those are just a few reminiscences of some nurses; there are many more untold and unwritten. The hope is that these have set your mind working, remembering both the good and the not so good times you had, during your training and afterwards. Perhaps it has woken some nostalgic feelings to return to work which, although hard, had its rewards. The rest of the book is devoted to how you can achieve this and what you might expect, as seen through the eyes of those who have made that journey.

Further reading

Books

Bell, C. (Ed.) (1984) *Social Researching: Politics, Problems, Practice.* Routledge & Kegan Paul, London.

Dingwall, R., Rafferty, A-M. & Webster, C. (1988) *Introduction to Social History of Nursing.* Routledge, London.

Hutter, B. & Williams, G. (1981) *Controlling Women. The Normal and the Deviant.* Croom Helm, London.

White, R. (Ed.) (1986) *Political Issues in Nursing. Volume 2. Past, Present and Future.* Wiley, Chichester.

Articles

Summers, A. (1989) The Mysterious Demise of Sarah Gamp: The Domiciliary Nurse and her Detractors. *Journal of Victorian Studies,* **32** 365–86. Leicester University.

Chapter 2
The Interim Years

Lack of confidence

One factor almost all nurses have in common when they have been out of practice for some years, is a lack of confidence. This usually bears no relation to the number of years out of nursing or to the position they held prior to leaving their last job.

Hutter & Williams (1981) (see Further Reading) suggested that lack of recent training or work experience serves to decrease self-esteem and may even limit the ability to perform competently. This lack of self-esteem could also be a result of the role of the sexes in the socialization practices which still operate within our society. When it is convenient, for example, at times of high unemployment, society holds the view that the mother should be in the home when the children are young. Indeed time and again nurses state that their reason for remaining at home so long, out of practice, is to care for their children.

Historically our culture has mandated that men work outside the home while women have a choice of joining the workforce or remaining within the home. While many women have to work outside the home because of economic need, the married, middle class, non-practising nurse may not need to work for financial reasons.

However, although this traditional role of women may indicate that many non-practising nurses feel they need to be in the home, their lifestyle demonstrates that they are engaged in many activities outside the home. These may range from some form of paid employment, not necessarily connected directly to nursing, through voluntary work to social pastimes and studying. During the course of these activities individuals will have accumulated a range of knowledge and skills which they will bring with them when they return to nursing.

This is demonstrated by the letter of application written by Mary Simmonds, a returning nurse, when applying for a part-time staff nurse post:

'I am at present employed as a playgroup assistant at Kidlington Playgroup. The playgroup provides a safe environment where children of three to five years old can learn from a wide range of experiences not always available at home. They learn through play about number, quantity, pre-reading and writing, physical activities and music as well as co-operation and trust of other adults and children.

Playgroups also provide support and learning opportunities for both parents and teenagers who come for work experience. I have been associated with the playgroup for ten years as parent, committee member, including chairman and secretary, voluntary helper and paid helper since 1982. I was a founder member of the Kidlington branch of the Pre-School Playgroups Association and attended a Playgroup Foundation Course run by the branch.

I have been a member of Kidlington Evening Townswomen's Guild for many years and take an active part in all the Guild's activities. I have been secretary of the executive committee and am still on the committee as social studies chairman which involves arranging outings and visits for both recreational and educational purposes.

I belong to the Kidlington Amateur Operatic Society and take an active part in concerts and in stage productions. I have recently been elected to the committee as secretary.

I have many other interests including reading, dressmaking, knitting, creative embroidery and gardening.'

Life experiences

One often reads in books and articles that the mature person brings 'life experiences' with them when they return to work. Presumably these experiences had not occurred when the individual left work and it is implied that they are desirable assets which will enhance the person's performance in the workplace.

If we accept that we are as a person what we have learned so far, we should be able to describe ourselves in terms of what we have learned, i.e. what we know, how we behave and how we react to situations. However, education is more than just an initiation into new fields of activity; it is a lifelong process. It follows that an educated person is one whose range of actions, reactions and activities are gradually transformed by the deepening and widening of understanding and sensitivity.

If we apply some of these beliefs about learning to some of the more common activities women and men have been involved in during the years they have been out of nursing, it should be possible to identify some experiences which have particular relevance to nursing practice today. These should indicate that, far from lacking knowledge and skills, returners have in fact enriched and added to their ability to function at a high level of skill.

'Nurturing'

Although to a large extent ill-defined, the central practices of women in the home might include the rearing of children, the education of children and adults, care of the dying, nursing the sick and injured and a variety of activities related to daily life such as cooking, washing, cleaning, gardening and shopping. These practices are sometimes described as 'nuturing', and as such carry a low status and are thought to be unskilled.

This is not to suggest that women are doing a variety of mindless tasks in response to the demands of others, rather it should be recognized that creativity and responsibility is required to conduct the practices to the full.

Housework

It is often assumed that women are natural homemakers and have acquired the knowledge and skills required to function efficiently and effectively in the home. It is also assumed that a woman enjoys and obtains a great deal of satisfaction and fulfilment from this work.

Perhaps because housework is considered to be a 'natural', unskilled, unspecific and unspecifiable activity with boundaries that shift constantly, it has never been highly regarded as a recommendation in the open labour market. Women themselves will say, when asked what they do, 'Oh, I am *only* a housewife and/or mother', as if it was of no account and the easiest thing in the world to be. A deeper exploration of the complexities of managing a home and caring for the family will reveal some of the knowledge and skills required by the homemaker, which will be of value as she returns to nursing.

Childcare

Pregnancy and childbirth are unique experiences which can give the midwife an understanding and empathy with other women undergoing similar experiences. Childcare, too, enhances one's knowledge and understanding of the normal developmental stages as the child grows and matures. There is a need to know about the normal bodily functions such as feeding, eliminating and sleeping and how these change as the child develops. An understanding is required about childhood illnesses and how many of these can now be prevented by such things as immunization and by providing the right environment in which to grow. If a child is handicapped in any way, quite specific knowledge may be required to cope with the handicap.

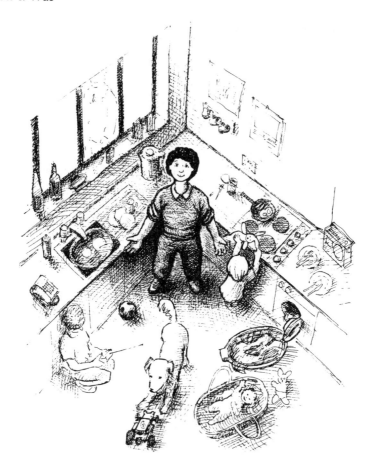

Unspecified, unspecifiable work.

One returning nurse recounted how the experience of caring for her own son who died of leukaemia was put to good use when caring for a boy and his family who were coping with similar problems. She was able not only to deal with the day to day problems but could also anticipate their future need for care and support.

The skills required in childcare may range from the basic ones of washing, feeding and changing the small baby to the training required to make a child socially acceptable in terms of eating, eliminating, playing and working with other children and adults. In addition there is a need at various times to be a teacher, a trainer, a counsellor, a listener, an advisor, a diplomat and an advocate.

Many of the above skills were needed by a returning nurse working in the Accident and Emergency Department when a cot death baby was brought in. As the only mother among the staff on duty she was delegated to sit with the distraught mother in Sister's office. The nurse recalls:

'After introducing myself, we sat for some time without speaking. I then asked the mother if she would like a cup of tea or coffee. Her reply startled me; all she wanted was to hold her baby. I knew there was no need for discussion; it was an important stage in her mourning to really believe her child was indeed dead. I also knew this might prove difficult for the staff to understand and agree to. They were however quite willing to wrap the baby up and give her to me to take to the mother.

Our nerves were tested to the limit when the mother kept the baby for five hours, through the visit of her pastor, husband, older children and social worker. She then voluntarily returned the baby into my arms. Although a harrowing experience for all the staff, I was possibly the one with the skills best able to cope with the situation, offering comfort and support to the family and the staff.'

Care of the elderly

It is often assumed by society in general and elderly people in particular that as they become increasingly frail a female relative will care for them. She will be expected to act, usually in a voluntary capacity, as a source of physical and social support for not only the elderly but also the physically and mentally handicapped.

It has been estimated that three times more old people live with their married daughters than with their married sons. In many instances this will curtail any activity the woman might want to participate in outside the home, including paid work. Such a situation was graphically described to me by one nurse wanting to return to work but wondering if she could manage. She explained that she cares for an 86-year-old aunt who is quite dependent on her.

'You come into it very gradually. At first she (the aunt) could not manage her shopping so I would pop in each day to see if she wanted anything. Then her home showed signs of neglect, so a little housework was added to the daily visit. Then washing and cooking needed to be included and it was just taken for granted by everyone that I would do it all. Now she is so dependent I cannot back out and leave her, especially as she is so desperate to stay in her own place. Then my father-in-law suffered a severe stroke. As he is widowed and lives alone it was decided that he should be placed in a nursing home. I must admit I was secretly thankful but I also feel very guilty when we visit him and he makes it quite plain that he would prefer to be in his own home!'

When I asked this nurse what knowledge and skills she thought she had acquired through these experiences it was difficult at first for her to single out anything specific. On reflection however she felt that she had acquired a deeper understanding of the ageing process and how one can lose one's independence either slowly, faculty by faculty, as with her aunt, or suddenly and catastrophically as with her father-in-law.

She felt she has also developed a knowledge of available resources in her locality, either to maintain the elderly in their own homes or to care for those who need expert care as in a nursing home. As she has taken on more care of her aunt she has had to learn to identify needs, set priorities and plan care, and fit these into her already busy life.

She has had to develop her communication and interpersonal skills in dealing with both her aunt and father-in-law and in negotiating with the professionals with whom they come into contact. She also realized when her father-in-law became dependent that there was a limit to her ability to cope and she was able, albeit reluctantly, to say a firm no to having him back home to be cared for by the family. All these are useful attributes to bring with her as she returns to nursing.

Homemaker

Motherhood and care of the elderly and disabled are usually taken on by women in addition to, not as a simplification of, their normal home care responsibilities. It is expected that the homemaker, whether male or female, will produce nutritious, nourishing meals when required, to suit individual tastes, food fads and fashions. It is assumed that the homemaker has the knowledge and skills to do this quite complicated task and has failed if unable to meet this basic human need.

From childhood most girls and a few boys are taught how and what to cook for themselves and others. Sometimes nutritional values and dietary needs are included in the knowledge base but this information could well be confused and clouded by a plethora of books, articles and television programmes which offer conflicting advice and suggestions. It is left to the individual to find her own way towards a healthy diet for herself and her family. This may be guided more by what the family likes, what they can afford and what can be easily prepared, rather than advice from the so-called experts.

One returning nurse, a mother, persuaded the hospital where she worked to introduce jacket potatoes and wholemeal bread to the menu, to the delight of patients and staff and possibly to the benefit of their health.

Financial manager

Closely linked with the provision of meals is the issue of budgeting. For most people the skills required to manage money are not necessarily part of their normal upbringing. They have in the past usually only had their own often small income to deal with, deciding what their priorities are from one wage packet to the next. On marriage they will be expected with little or no help to manage a budget for eventually several people, often with only one source of income. They must assess the needs of the individuals, decide their priorities and look for the best value for money. There are very few families who escape the struggle of trying to get a quart out of a pint pot.

The skills of being able to manage on a limited income were seldom required from nurses in the past. Today however, most nurse managers will be expected to keep within a limited budget for staff and supplies. They will need to prioritize not only on cost but also on moral and ethical grounds. Can they afford to employ a bank or agency nurse or do they close some beds knowing that somebody will suffer as a result? Is one dressing more effective than another? Should they order it even though it is going to cost more?

One returning nurse was on the receiving end of such decisions recently. She could only work on a casual basis at her local hospital. This worked well initially when she had all the work she could manage. But when the hospital ran out of money in its nursing budget they could no longer afford to employ her, even though they still needed her services. It was a hard decision for both of them.

Technology and equipment

There is no doubt that the technological revolution which has descended on the workplace has also intruded to some degree into the home. If the statistics are to be believed it is now commonplace to find a refrigerator, washing machine and carpet cleaner in most households. Add to these the cookers, food preparation equipment and microwaves in the kitchen and television, video machines and hi-fi sound equipment in the lounge of a high proportion of households, and it can easily be seen that the modern housewife, even if she only owns a few of these devices, can no longer be afraid of technology in general. She has had to learn how to manage often quite complicated machinery in order to get the best value from it, and to be persuaded that it can do the job more effectively and efficiently than she can.

Nursing, which is quite labour intensive, can be greatly enhanced by the use of technology, providing improved patient care and freeing the nurse from boring, repetitive jobs. Monitoring equipment, ward laboratory testing of blood, urine and faeces, apparatus to assist with patient mobility can all help the nurse in her care of patients, but must be mastered first by anyone using them. Returning nurses should not fear technology but should see it as an aid to their care.

Information technology

Another rapidly growing field of technology, both in the home and in nursing, is information technology. Advertisers would suggest that our lives are about to be taken over by computers. Many households with school age children have already been persuaded to purchase computers with games and more sophisticated packages which can manage a whole range of activities from word processing to desk-top publishing, from making simple calculations to ordering the weekly groceries.

It would appear that as we move through the 1990s, technology will for most of us become a part of normal daily living. More and more hospitals, health authorities and general practitioners are setting up computer-linked systems for storing and retrieving patient data. Nurses too are learning to use computers to record information and to use data already recorded by others.

Business manager

For some women, as their children grow older and become less demanding, work outside the home becomes a real possibility. For many a quite natural progression is to help in their husband's business. This help might range from simply answering the telephone, responding to queries and taking orders, to being on the board of directors if the business is larger and more sophisticated.

The skills and knowledge required for such diverse and varied activities will depend on the particular business concerned and the amount of involvement. For example, most farmers' wives will need a working knowledge of and skills in animal husbandry and/or crop management. Many take a course in book-keeping as few small farmers can afford the luxury of skilled secretarial help. They will be used to long, unsociable hours and hard, physical work, often with poor rewards. They will sometimes be accustomed to delivering and hand rearing farm livestock and perhaps working a range of farm machinery. Their work could well be seasonal and they become used to flexible and adaptable working hours and conditions.

Although much of this work can find a direct parallel with nursing, one ward did have a problem with a returning nurse who had a small livestock farm. When she was asked if she would be happy giving an injection, she replied in a loud voice in the hearing of the patient that she had that week injected a hundred sheep.

General practitioners' wives also have to be prepared to be flexible and adaptable, especially if their husbands are not one of a larger practice. The wives expect to have to act in an emergency, whether on the telephone or on their doorstep, if the doctor is not around. Their ability to keep calm in a crisis and administer emergency first-aid is occasionally tested to the limit.

Interpersonal skills

From what most returning nurses tell me, if they have a husband who runs a family business – whether it is in production, retailing or a service – the wives will need to develop interpersonal skills to deal with the workforce and customers. Communication skills are also an absolute necessity when dealing with people, whether face to face, on the telephone or in writing. Social skills become important as the business builds up, with a need to entertain clients and recruit and retain staff.

All these skills are also needed by women who have set up their own business, often as a result of dissatisfaction or desperation with the local provision. One nurse told me that she became so disillusioned with the nursing agency she joined that she felt sure she could run one more efficiently. With a friend she set up and successfully ran her own. She insisted that her nurses were of a high standard and were only allocated to work she thought they could manage.

Another nurse found that she was unable to nurse because there was no local nursery or playgroup provision, so she set up her own playschool. Both these businesses were successful and were only given up because the nurses moved on.

The management experience gained either running or helping to run a business will prove invaluable in nursing today. Handling personnel, training, problem solving, and decision making are all skills required by the modern nurse who is more likely to give total care to a group of patients than follow orders giving care to all the patients on a ward.

Voluntary work

Apart from the unpaid voluntary work women do in their own homes, either caring for elderly and handicapped relatives or helping their husbands pursue their own business, they are often fair game as 'unemployed' women to take on some voluntary responsibility for the community in which they live. This work might include the following:

(1) *Aide*   Helping out on a casual or regular basis in the local nursery or primary school as a teachers' aide, listening to children learning to read, supervising a cookery group or helping with a games lesson.
(2) *Chauffeur*   Using the car to ferry people around to the doctor's surgery, to the local hospital, shopping, visiting, assisting with meals on wheels and the mobile library for the housebound, and participating in the school run.

(3) *Committee person*   Being drawn into committee work in a variety of capacities, from secretary to treasurer, from chairman to caterer, for a range of charity or voluntary organizations.
(4) *Political work*   Becoming involved in political groups, either as a participant serving officer in local or national government or as a governor in public service such as schools, colleges or the health service.

Although many of these activities might seem trivial on an individual basis, they do tend to accumulate and are usually quite important to the person who has accepted that responsibility. One woman who found it difficult to say no became ill as a result of her responsibilities. She already had a full time job yet she was also secretary of two local women's groups, treasurer to a charity, a member of the Conservative Club, a committee member of the local tennis club, and was also responsible for arranging the flowers in her local church each week.

It is difficult to be specific in identifying the skills and knowledge required for the above activities. They all differ in character and depth of responsibility, yet there is some common ground covering many of the activities. There are obvious skill areas such as interpersonal, communication and driving. Less obvious or common might be the need for teaching, secretarial, organizational and management skills. A working knowledge of financial matters, local and national government, voluntary agencies and the educational and health systems will be needed by those involved in particular activities.

A willingness to be adaptable and flexible to cope with the ever-changing world and the effect this will have on the local community, and a preparedness to fight to retain vital resources, especially in remote communities, become part of the character of the 'unemployed' member of that community. These characteristics were exemplified by the account of one returning nurse who, when asked what she had brought back into nursing with her, gave the following account:

'I was invited to join a group discussion about the discharge of an elderly male patient who had suffered a severe stroke. Discussion centred around his medical condition and its possible prognosis. It was agreed that he needed regular physiotherapy and some specialized equipment to assist his independence at home. As the only mature nurse present it was I who pointed out the domestic and social problems of this man. He lived in a small, isolated village with an elderly wife and there were few facilities in the community to help them, such as local transport or shops or even neighbours with free time. Hospital staff seem unaware or not even to care whether on discharge patients will be able to cope with normal daily activities of living.'

Paid employment

Of course not all women at home can afford the luxury of participating in unpaid voluntary work; they need to have some income, no matter how small, to swell the family budget. Some form of nursing work will not be an option either because of the difficulties with transport if they live in a rural area, or because their domestic circumstances prevent them from committing themselves to regular hours.

The non-nursing work which people become involved in is very varied ranging from temporary positions such as research assistant for a marketing or drug company, to casual work in a bank or secretarial agency, or work in the local primary or nursery school as classroom assistant or playground supervisor or dinner lady.

Many other part-time occupations have been mentioned by individual returners, such as shop or factory work, cleaning and catering, hairdressing and beauty therapist, and counsellor.

It would be difficult to identify what the individuals gained from their work experiences as these are so wide and varied. But as mentioned earlier, education is a lifelong process and most people will have gained in maturity, sensitivity and understanding and will be more able to empathize with their patients when they talk about the effect their illness will have either in continuing the same job or looking for alternative work. One nurse recalls an incident with a patient which illustrates this:

'I was helping to bath a man in his sixties, who had suffered a stroke. As I was drying him he asked me if I would cut his toe nails. They had not been attended to for several weeks, so I looked for the ward's nail-clippers. They were nowhere to be found so, because of the patient's obvious distress, I sacrificed my own surgical scissors. As I trimmed his nails he told me how important his feet were to him and how particular he had always been in cutting his nails and ensuring he had good shoes. What was his occupation? A postman!'

Studying

More and more mothers are using the interim years, while their children are growing up, to study either for interest or more often to gain further qualifications in the expectation that these will be of benefit when they return to work. The courses undertaken and the qualifications gained vary enormously. They may range from City and Guilds

Embroidery I and II to a history degree, from shorthand and typing to a teaching qualification.

Some find they can only manage courses by distance or open learning, with or without tutorial support. Whatever the course content and outcome all will have gained experience in study skills and in the discipline needed to pursue a learning experience through to completion. Success will also bring an increase in confidence and self esteem which will encourage the individual to seek further educational development. This will be a considerable asset in nursing today where nurses have a professional responsibility to increase and develop their own knowledge and skills and share them with their peers and subordinates.

Overseas travel

Nurses who have travelled abroad and gained experience nursing in other countries have acquired and developed invaluable knowledge and skills. Coping with different cultures and learning a new language while adapting one's own training to suit local circumstances, requires considerable flexibility and adaptability. Safely cocooned in the National Health Service or private medicine in this country it is difficult for us to imagine the difficulties and privations nurses and patients elsewhere have to suffer, especially in third world countries. Yet as this country becomes increasingly multi-racial there is a growing need for nurses to not only understand the language but also the cultural differences which affect the care they offer patients and the patients' interpretation of that care. A nurse from Nigeria made the following observations after working in this country for a few months:

> 'Nigerian hospitals suffer from chronic under-funding, with the resultant shortage of basic equipment. One never discarded anything if another use could be found for it. For example, empty intravenous fluid bags were used to collect urine and wound drainage. I am appalled at the wastage in this country. In Nigeria doctors would write out prescriptions and relatives would have to buy the drug from the local pharmacy if they could afford it. If they had no money the patient went without the drug. Even oxygen could be in short supply, a situation which led to tragedy for one baby who died because there was no more oxygen available that night. Average life expectancy in Nigeria is about 60 years for men and women. This means that elderly care is almost non-existent. Active treatment in hospital was usually focused almost exclusively on young people. One notable exception was severely handicapped babies who seldom survived.'

Nurses who have worked abroad have learned not to make hurried judgements about people or conditions, but to see them in context and understand why situations have developed in a certain way. They have acquired a depth of maturity not easily understood or appreciated by those who have not enjoyed that experience. Working in remote stations hundreds of miles from civilization, whether it is with Eskimos in Northern Canada, primitive tribes in the African bush or Aborigines in the Australian outback, the nurses have to fall back on their own resources using a mixture of experience, intuition and expertise. This is not always accepted by nurses in this country, as the Nigerian nurse recalled:

'I was caring for an elderly man with a chronic chest condition. I just knew he was about to arrest. When I asked for the arrest team my colleagues laughed and sent me off for a meal break. When I returned the patient was dead. I explained that in my country we only had one anaesthetist, who carried the resuscitation equipment with him. We therefore learned to detect very early any symptoms of distress.'

Leisure activities

For any nurse, leisure time pursuits help to enrich and develop the individual personality. Returning nurses are engaged in a whole range of activities from sport to the arts, both participating and organizing. Many of these pursuits and talents can be utilized to the benefit of patients. Two main areas that spring to mind are rehabilitation and fund raising for patient benefits. There is a much stronger emphasis today on encouraging patients to become as independent as possible, adapting their activities within the range of their capabilities. This is often achieved through leisure activities such as games involving skill and chance through to more purposeful activities such as knitting, sewing, gardening, painting and woodwork. Many nurses will become involved in these activities with patients, often in their own time, building up a relationship as they share a common interest.

In one elderly care unit a nurse who had shown an interest in and ability for leisure pursuits was appointed part-time leisure activity co-ordinator and spent most afternoons working with patients on a planned programme of activities ranging from ballroom or sequence dancing to handicrafts. These were designed to strengthen weak muscles and ease stiff joints and also build up confidence and self esteem. Many hand-made and home grown items are sold to defray the cost of production and supplement the funds of the unit.

Nursing is a demanding, complex job requiring a range of abilities to give continuity and safe care around the clock. In order to function effectively a nurse needs:

- Well developed skills of communication.
- A great sensitivity.
- A good degree of manual dexterity.
- A sound knowledge base.
- The ability to be flexible and adaptable.
- The ability to teach individually and in small groups.
- Managerial knowledge and expertise.
- A willingness to co-operate and work in a team.
- An ability to use her own initiative.

The newly qualified nurse might possess many of these but in a rudimentary form. The nurse who is out of practice for a number of years will have enhanced and developed her mastery of many skills, bringing about an improvement in her performance.

Further reading

Books

Brion, M. & Tinker, A. (1980) *Women in Housing.* Housing Centre Trust. Open University.

Brown, J.K. & Kerns, V. (1985) *In Her Prime.* Bergin & Garvey, Massachusetts.

Hutter, B. & Williams, G. (1981) *Controlling Women. The Normal and the Deviant.* Croom Helm, London.

Lawson, K.H. (1989) *Philosophical Concepts in Adult Education.* Oxford University Press.

Peters, R.S. & Dray, W.H. (1975) *The Philosophy of Education.* Oxford University Press.

Rogers, C. (1986 reprint) *On Becoming a Person.* Constable, London.

Articles

James, N. (1989) Emotional Labour: Skill and Work in the Social Regulation of Feelings. *Sociological Review,* **37**(1) 15–42. Routledge.

Kitson, A. (1987) A Comparative Analysis of Long-Caring and Professional (Nursing) Caring Relationships. *International Journal of Nursing Studies,* **24**(2) 155–65.

Part 2
Time to Return

Chapter 3
Why Return?

Rediscovering past experiences and assessing their quality and meaning is an important step towards personal and professional development and rejoining the job market. The next step is to utilize that knowledge and awareness to set personal goals from the wide range of choices available. It is important that people recognize their own capabilities, take opportunities and take responsibility for their own futures.

In real life most decisions involve a complex interplay of many factors; anything or everything can help make up one's mind. What therefore motivates a nurse to return to nursing after some years away could be anything from the need for personal development and growth to the more mundane need for money and security.

Reasons for returning

Need for money

One of the most powerful and frequently mentioned motives for returning to nursing today is the need for money. In today's financial climate this is hardly surprising; with the burden of mortgage repayments and interest rates plus the expense of rearing a family, few families can manage for more than one or two years on one source of income. There is also a rising number of one-parent families who are otherwise often dependent on the state for all their financial needs. Most women returning to the job market first explore the possibility of returning to the work with which they were familiar when they left to raise their family. Ex-nurses will therefore look to the possibility of returning to nursing, usually on a part-time or casual basis. With the current level of nurse's salary this can be quite lucrative as one nurse discovered:

> 'I do one night a week on "D" grade and take home £50. Keeping to this amount I manage to stay outside the tax and National Insurance brackets so I keep all the money I earn. If I worked two nights it

would cost me more than the disruption to the family is worth. With one night I can manage without any support, even during the school holidays. I am surprised more nurses have not discovered this. It also helps to keep me in touch.'

Night duty and unsociable hours are of course paid at an enhanced rate at the moment and if the post is a permanent one rather than casual work, the nurse will be entitled to paid holidays and incremental increases in salary.

Becoming single

Next to the need for money, and perhaps inextricably linked with it, the death of or divorce from one's partner is a strong motivator for returning to the workforce. Some return willingly and with a sense of relief:

> 'My husband, James, died two years ago after a long illness. I decided to return to nursing a year ago and found it an excellent therapy. After many years away from the profession my knees knocked somewhat, and many things were different, but I have settled down and found myself part of a happy team.'

Others however might feel resentful that due to circumstances beyond their control they are being forced into resuming work from necessity rather than choice. It has been known for solicitors in divorce cases to ring the local hospital to check whether the nurse can return to the workforce. I recently interviewed a divorced woman who explained why she was enquiring about returning to nursing:

> 'I have been divorced for eleven years and out of nursing for fourteen years. I have a non-nursing job now which is full time and which I enjoy very much. Unfortunately it is poorly paid with no chance of any great increase either in money or hours. I have just received a letter from my solicitor informing me that in four years time when my son leaves school all maintenance will stop from my ex-husband and I will have to keep myself. If I returned to nursing I could double the salary that I receive currently in my non-nursing work. I do not particularly want to return to nursing, but it looks as if I have no choice.'

On the positive side however a newspaper report suggested recently that divorced women returning to work are more likely to make a success of their career than divorced men who remain in the same job.

Boredom

Boredom is another powerful oft-quoted reason for returning to the workforce, particularly after the children have started school or left home. The 'empty nest' syndrome causes many women to re-evaluate their lives and consider what they want to achieve. Some women will want to explore areas of career and vocational interest which will add to an understanding of themselves, the health care environment and the larger world of work. Others say they have no real idea of what they want to do, but they have been talking about returning to work for a long time so they will start first and then decide later on what it is they really want to do. One nurse, who admitted to being bored at home, reflected after her first day of a Return to Nursing course:

'As I made my way home I felt alive. Even though the day was physically and mentally tiring, it was at the same time stimulating. I suddenly felt important as a person. I was called by my christian name; I had almost forgotten what it sounded like. It was great to mix with and talk to people with similar problems and experiences. It was a strange feeling, too, to have others think you had something important to say and that you had something to offer which was valued. I realised I was now entering a world which did not directly involve either my family or the community in which I lived.'

Nostalgia

Nostalgia plays a part in encouraging some nurses to return to work. This is often triggered by direct contact with a hospital, either as a patient or as a visitor helping to care for a close family member or friend. This gives the time and opportunity to observe what is happening at close quarters and compare it with past experience, and this may convince the nurse that they are still capable of picking up the threads of their old career. On the other hand some are so enraged by what they see as poor standards of care that they want to return to put things right, as illustrated by the following account:

'I recently spent three weeks at . . . hospital. Not a very pleasant experience. Not once did I see the senior nurse or anyone else in administration. Nursing is certainly not what it was, and after my stay in hospital I am only too thankful I trained years ago. Mobilization is the watchword now, no matter how the patient feels. There is too much 'personal' chatter over the patient's bed and the constant cry 'I'll be back in a minute', which invariably becomes hours. The weeks I spent in a small cottage hospital convalescing were much happier.'

Guilt

Nurses out of practice are often made to feel guilty for not using the knowledge and skills they have. Television, radio and newspapers exploit to the full the local and national problems in the National Health Service and in nursing. The media emphasize the need to close beds, wards and hospitals, and how many operations are cancelled causing patients to be turned away, thus lengthening the waiting lists. The shortage of qualified nurses is the reason given for many of these calamities. It comes as a surprise therefore to nurses who respond to such appeals, to discover perhaps that the shortages are confined to a few local hospitals, not in their own locality, or the shortage is in highly specialized units such as intensive care or special baby units requiring highly specialized, skilled nurses.

'Pushed into' a return

The general public, and to some extent the professions allied to nursing, believe in the 'generic' nurse. They believe that a nurse can carry out the role of a nurse in any given circumstance, e.g. a friend or neighbour asking for advice and help on what to do about a range of health problems from a cut or bee sting to a medical emergency. People are unaware of the growing specialization in nursing which requires a high level of knowledge and skills, acquired usually through an advanced course, to care for a particular group of patients such as those in renal dialysis and transplant units, those being anaesthetized, those in plastic surgery units and so on.

This general misunderstanding of what nursing is today is reflected in the number of nurses who are pushed back into the workforce by well-meaning people. Frequently mentioned in this context are the local general practitioner and the local vicar or priest. They seem to see nursing as a panacea for many emotional or domestic problems, not realizing that this might exacerbate the situation rather than improve it.

It is my experience also that if someone's heart is not really in their work they will eventually leave for something else, as illustrated by the following account from a tutor:

'Many years ago I was approached by a Catholic priest about one of his congregation. She had moved south with her two teenage daughters about five years previously, after the death of her husband. She knew no one in the area where she settled but quite unexpectedly she met a man who eventually proposed marriage to her. As her daughters were on the point of leaving home to pursue their careers and she feared being alone, she agreed to marry him. Before this event took place he collapsed and died, leaving her absolutely devastated. In an effort to help her the priest, who discovered she used to be a nurse – albeit 20 or more years ago – had the bright idea of getting her back into nursing.

I agreed to help but this was before courses were run for this purpose, so the help had to be individually organized with a mixture of classroom instruction and clinical support over many months. She then worked part-time for about two years. I never really felt that her heart was in the work. So it was no surprise to me, when I met her recently, to be told that she had left nursing and was pursuing a very different career in local government.'

Reasons for not returning

Fear

Just as strong as the many reasons for returning to nursing are the diverse and original reasons for not returning to the workforce. These may range from trying to come to terms with working and running a home to low self esteem coupled with lack of child care provision. But underlying most of these reasons is the need to confront and overcome the widespread fear that most people experience when faced with the return to work. The causes of this fear may range from a general feeling of inadequacy brought about from being out of the workforce for a number of years, to a fear of making a fool of oneself in front of colleagues through a lack of knowledge or skills in an area of work where one had some expertise many years ago. Or, as one returning nurse said when enquiring about a returners course:

'I don't want to appear as a bumbling old person to the young, more recently qualified nurses.'

Developments in drugs

Another very real fear nurses have is the lack of recent training which may limit their ability to perform competently. The recent rapid advances in health care and changes in nursing serve to make the returner feel their basic preparation is now obsolete.

Drugs are often quoted in this context. The worry that many new drugs are now on the market which can be potent, and the publicity given to accidental overdoses, compound the anxiety nurses feel. What they do not appreciate however is that this fear is recognized and understood in nursing today, leading to safer systems of work being introduced so that returners should not be involved with drug administration until they feel ready.

Also, drug rounds of all the patients on the ward are becoming less

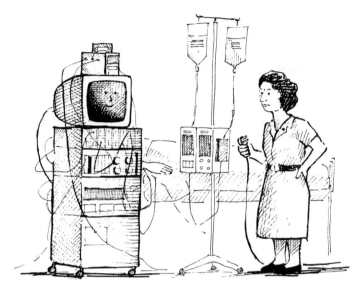

How does this work?

common. Nurses are much more likely to give drugs only to the group of patients they are caring for. In addition, information about drugs is much more readily available in an understandable form, and pharmacists are only too willing to be consulted if a problem or misunderstanding arises on the ward.

Technical equipment

Because medical technology, such as monitoring, giving IV injections and pumps and sealed drainage, is very evident to anyone walking on to an acute hospital ward – and nowadays is even found in some homes – nurses out of work have the impression that care is impossible without using seemingly highly technical equipment.

The ability to use a new tool or piece of equipment skilfully should not be minimized, but it needs to be put into the proper perspective of the work as a whole. Equipment is continually changing and most nurses can learn to use simple equipment by reading the instructions. As mentioned in Chapter 2, a majority of homes in the UK possess some piece of technology designed to assist or enhance home life, and this needed to be mastered to become effective. In the workplace more complicated equipment requires on-the-job training for any nurse. Yet even with such training obvious gaps exist, allowing nurses to make mistakes. This is demonstrated by one returning nurse who assumed that a bed pan masher was a bed pan washer:

'She had been out of nursing for 14 years and this was the first time she had come across disposable bedpans. She put a plastic pan in the masher and forever after was known as "Masher Haydon". How easy it is to forget that nurses returning to the profession are not up to date with present day gadgets.' Quoted from a project by M. Mavroleon (1989). (See Further Reading.)

But returning nurses should not let such disposables and equipment present an insurmountable barrier to their return to active nursing. Rather they should see how they might work faster and with less frustration than they formerly knew with older methods.

Family responsibilities

Home and family responsibilities present many prospective returning nurses with seemingly impossible difficulties in their quest to rejoin the workforce. Problems arise from trying to fulfil the role obligations and normal aspects of all relationships in addition to the demands of a job. In an effort to make the whole system manageable the returner must decide how to allocate her energies and skills so as to make working a possibility.

Husbands are not always as helpful and co-operative as they might be. This attitude may stem from their mixed feelings about the perceived loss of their wife and housekeeper and the usurping of their role as sole provider for the family. Most husbands still assume that their work is of prime importance and everything else must therefore fit around them, rather than them making allowances for a working wife. It is important therefore that the returner involves her husband in the decision to return to work.

Other family members will also need to be included in the discussions. They will need to understand the implications of the decreased availability of the mother and the need for them all to assume additional responsibilities in the home and make commitments to be supportive. But the reality of trying to juggle with the demands of a family and career may well lead to conflict eventually, as one returner experienced:

'I have a semi-invalid husband and four children in their early teens. We discussed my return to work fully, I thought, and agreed on sharing out some of my responsibilities in the home. All went well at first; we all appreciated having more money and I felt more fulfilled and interesting as a person. Slowly, almost imperceptibly, I gradually resumed more and more of the household chores. I tried not to be a nagging wife and mother but became increasingly angry that I was expected not only to work but also to carry out the household duties.

One Sunday morning things came to a head when I found myself not only cooking the Sunday lunch single-handed but also cleaning out the family car, which I did not drive, while the family were indulging in their own pastimes. Sunday lunch spoiled that day while we sorted out again our individual responsibilities, with the ultimatum that if it did not work this time the alternative was for me to stay at home and not go out to work.'

Childcare provision

One of the greatest difficulties women have to overcome when re-turning to work is childcare provision, and sometimes provision for care of elderly relatives. For most women family responsibilities must take priority over work commitments. Many state that they chose to have children, therefore it is their duty to care for them. It is important that any prospective employer has a clear understanding that family responsibilities exist and ascertains what provision is made for them.

Although the returning nurse will try to anticipate every eventuality, difficulties may well arise which could not be foreseen. These may range from health problems, such as minor coughs and colds, major trauma or serious illness, to a breakdown in childcare provision such as the childminder withdrawing or the closure of nursery, crèche or play-group facilities in the locality. It is important therefore that the returning nurse considers carefully the difficulties that might arise and the pro-vision she might make to overcome them.

It has been well documented and discussed in a variety of forums that the major problem mothers face in returning to work is the lack of childminding facilities available in this country. Only a fortunate few families have nearby grandparents or family members who can care for their young children whether they are pre-school age or just require supervision during school holidays.

Some employers, including Health Authorities, recognize the need to provide a nursery and childminding service during school holidays to enable nurses to return to work earlier than would otherwise be possible. These provisions however are often costly, both for the employer and employee, and have only limited usefulness. The hours the provision is available and the age groups they accept do not always meet the requirements of individual users.

One returning nurse was offered a permanent post as a district nurse which she would have loved to accept both for professional satisfaction and personal development. She was forced however to decline the offer for family reasons.

She has two boys, aged 8 and 11 years, who attend different schools. This means they finish school at different times and school holidays do not always coincide. They are too young to be left at home unattended, yet object to having childminders. Their father cannot help with their care so the mother has to be there when they are at home. This means that in order to maintain her nursing skills she is obliged to work on a casual basis for the nurse bank. This she will have to do for at least another five years.

Understanding motivation

Understanding what motivates or demotivates an individual nurse, in returning to the workforce, is important not only for the nurse but also for the manager. The provision of 'in touch' and Return to Nursing courses, flexible working patterns and part-time work which encourages professional development, must all become part of employment strategy. Positive attitudes to create an environment that enables a nurse to feel wanted and a valued member of the team, will encourage a returner who may be unsure of her own worth in the current work market.

Further reading

Books

Buzan, T. (1982) *Use Your Head*. Ariel Books, London.

Castles, F.G. *et al.* (1976) *Decisions, Organisation and Society*. Oxford University Press.

Kagan, C., Evans, J. & Kay, B. (1986) *A Manual of Interpersonal Skills*. Harper & Row, London.

Paul, W.J. & Robertson, K.B. (1970) *Job Enrichment and Employee Motivation*. Gower, London.

Tschudin, V. & Scholer, J. (1990) *Managing Yourself*. Macmillan Education, London.

Articles

Curran, C.L. & Lengacher, C.A. (1982) RN [Registered Nurse] re-entry programmes: programmatic and personal considerations. *Nurse Educator*, **7**(3) 29–32.

Kelly, P.D. (1980) Low-cost Refresher Programmes. *Supervisor-Nurse*, **11**(7) 23.

Mavroleon, M. (1989) *The Second Time Around*. Unpublished project, Oxfordshire Health Authority.

Ruxton, J.P. (1981) Barriers to re-entry. Problems are many: solutions few. *California Nurse*, **77**(4) Sept/Oct.

Chapter 4
What Does Retraining Involve?

Currently there is a statutory requirement for only midwives to refresh periodically before they are allowed to practise as midwives. In theory no matter how many years a general trained nurse has been out of practice she can walk into any nursing job and practise her profession providing she has paid her fee and registered with the United Kingdom Central Council (UKCC). In practice however this can prove to be a terrifying experience, as recounted by two nurses who did just that.

The hard way

One nurse had been out of nursing for ten years and decided one day she would go round to her local cottage hospital to see if there was any work available, and what retraining they offered. She was told she would be given training as she went along and could she start that evening. This she did with no uniform, no contract and no health check.

She was working with another trained nurse who, because they were so busy, had neither the time nor patience to train what was, after all, a qualified nurse. The returning nurse felt like a fish out of water; she did not know what to do or how to do it. Many things had changed but one thing in particular she noticed: there was no longer an emphasis on basic nursing care. When she left work that evening she resolved to find out if there was some kind of retraining programme provided locally.

The second nurse had an even more horrifying experience. She had been out of nursing for 25 years, staying at home raising her children. She was taken on by an elderly care ward with the understanding that she would do the local retraining programme. Unfortunately that programme was cancelled so she had to wait five months for the next one to start; in the meantime she commenced work. When I asked her what it was like to walk on to a ward in a trained nurse's uniform, after 25 years, a look of sheer terror crossed her face as she said simply:

'It was horrendous. I felt a complete liability, no help at all. Physically I could cope with the work but mentally I felt so slow. It is

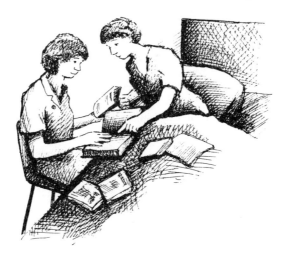

Just a minute, I'll read it up.

the little things which throw you, like you don't give daily blanket baths and it is not the nurse's job to wipe the lockers. The most frightening change is the accountability. You can no longer hide behind Sister's skirts as you did in the old days. I wish I was at least ten years younger and could have started work not wearing a trained nurse's uniform.'

Statutory retraining

Unfortunately these experiences are not unique and nurses up and down the country can relate similar stories. The UKCC has made it clear in its annual reports that it is committed to statutory up-date programmes for all nurses returning to nursing after a break of five years or more. It is highly likely that this will happen in the 1990s but there appears to be no national strategy for planning or implementing such programmes and certainly no extra funding identified for them. The UKCC issued guidelines of good practice for re-entry programmes in 1986 (see Fig. 4.1) but it is up to local Health Authorities to decide whether they follow these or even if they have a course at all. These requirements will be subject to revision once Return to Practise programmes become a statutory requirement.

In October 1988 the National Boards established a Return to Nursing Course in their Post Basic Nursing Studies Series. This is a fairly flexible, broad based course which 'shall be based in an approved training institution and shall be of 113 hours to 150 hours in length, half of which will be theoretical and half clinical/practical experience'. The outcomes of the course are closely related to the guidelines issued by the UKCC in 1986, mentioned above.

On completion of a 'Return to Practise Programme' the following outcomes which are based on up-to-date knowledge of the practice of nursing or health visiting should be achieved by the nurse, or health visitor:

3.1   an understanding of the current structure of health and social services, and resulting lines of authority and responsibility;

3.2   an understanding of appropriate current legislation, guidelines, codes of practice and policies;

3.3   an understanding of factors within the environment which relate to the safety of patients/clients, their families and colleagues;

3.4   the ability to design, execute and evaluate plans of patient/client care, based on appropriate models;

3.5   the ability to initiate and carry out emergency procedures effectively and as appropriate;

3.6   the ability to measure accurately, record and understand the relevance of patient/client data obtained by personal observation or through the use of equipment;

3.7   the ability to administer medicines safely;

3.8   the ability to use appropriate communciation skills in relation to patients/clients, relatives, and other members of the care team;

3.9   an understanding of the practitioner's educational role in relation to patients/clients, relations and colleagues.

3.10 an understanding of the current issues ànd training programmes which affect professional practice.

Fig. 4.1 Outcomes of Return to Practise programmes. (Source: Guidelines issued by UKCC.)

Availability of courses

For nurses seeking a retraining programme the news is not altogether inspiring. Availability will depend very much on where they live, how far they are prepared to travel, if they are willing to move house and in some instances how much they are prepared to pay. They will have to be highly motivated, persistent and not easily deterred from their objectives.

I have had nurses on my courses doing all these things in order to be retrained. Some have travelled over 50 miles each way to attend the theoretical sessions, but have often managed to do the practical work locally. At least two have moved home, renting local accommodation while their own houses are rented out to pay the mortgage. It took one nurse over a year of persistent enquiry to find my course and it entails her travelling 30 miles each way.

These are nurses who were determined to do a retraining programme before they took up paid employment as a qualified nurse. They also looked for the best possible course they could find and were not to be fobbed off with learning on the job or a few lectures on often unrelated topics.

Which course?

A whole range of people and organizations are now involved in running Return to Nursing courses. The type of course offered will depend on the demand and the resources available.

At one end of the range will be the local on-the-job induction/ orientation, provided by the staff in post who may be the ward sister or staff nurse with special responsibility in this area. It could be simply an introduction to the staff, ward layout and policies relating to the ward, or it might be more comprehensive and include nursing theory and medical information relating to the particular speciality.

Such on-the-job training might seem quite a sensible and attractive option, both to returning nurses and to nurse management. From the ward staff's point of view they have a willing recruit whom they can train in their own way in regard to organizing care and running the ward. From the nurses' point of view, they can quickly get back into the practical situation of earning money and have no particular need to do any studying other than that directly related to work.

The disadvantages of this method of retraining are that unless wards or departments make a conscious effort to keep their knowledge and practice in line with current thinking, the returning nurses might well be fed misinformation or inaccurate knowledge. They could also be taught unsafe practices if they have no other point of reference with which to make comparisons.

For the nurses this type of return to work is very limiting. It will prepare them to work in that work area or speciality only. They might feel inadequate if they moved into another area, but because they had already returned to work they might not be considered to be in need of further help. This could well create dissatisfaction in the returners, who would feel trapped in the areas in which they were working. Far from helping recruitment, on-the-job retraining could in fact become counter productive.

Induction/orientation programmes are important for anyone commencing employment in a new place but they cannot be seen as a substitute which will give any nurse the competence and confidence to resume fully the role of a qualified nurse. Returning nurses who have been out of practice for many years will need a course which not only understands their particular learning needs but also has the resources to meet those needs.

At the other end of the range of options for the returning nurse is a fully organized course run by an experienced highly qualified nurse teacher who preferably has post basic teaching experience. The teacher will also need the support and backing of an interested sympathetic management. Such courses may range from a one week full time residential course or a two hour evening class once a week for two academic terms, with no or optional clinical experience, to the nationally recognized English National Board (ENB) Return to Nursing course mentioned earlier.

Distance learning

More recently Open College in conjunction with the English National Board have produced a Return to Nursing course by distance learning. This involves working from work books, audio and video tapes. A network of action points has been set up throughout the country to facilitate the learner in using the package. Practical experience will have to be organized with the learner's local hospital, using the action point if possible.

Cost of courses

Most courses make a charge ranging from a modest £30 for the evening classes to several hundred pounds for the residential course. The fee will not usually cover the true cost of running such a course; the teacher's salary and overhead costs of heating, lighting and use of classrooms are absorbed by the department which runs the course. Similarly for the student the fee will represent only a small part of the expenses involved; child minding, travel, books, writing materials and professional registration fees and loss of earnings while studying will all add to the final costs.

Many people feel that in times of severe nursing shortage Health Authorities should not be charging for such courses but should be actually paying returners to attend them. It can be argued however that if Health Authorities are paying completely for the course, it is reasonable that they expect the returner to work for them at the end of the course. This assumes not only that jobs are available but that they are at times which are suitable for returners and in clinical areas where the returner wishes to work.

Another factor to be considered is that returners often attend a course to find out if, after all these years, they still want to return to nursing. If, as is sometimes the case, they find nursing is no longer the career they remembered, it is better to find out before making an expensive commitment.

Finally, people who run courses find that if a person has paid they will have far more motivation not only to attend regularly and complete the course but also to demand the best value for money.

It is possible for the organizers of Return to Nursing courses to obtain government funding to defray some of the costs, both for themselves and the students. This at the moment is called Employment Training and is money set aside by the government to retrain unemployed people to enable them to return to the workforce at little or no cost to themselves.

Need for a course

One factor that makes most returning nurses look for a suitable course is the lack of confidence they feel in their ability to nurse. Many are aware that changes have occurred, although they see those related more to practical concerns such as drugs, technology and procedures. They are afraid of making a mistake or being made to look foolish in front of colleagues or patients.

When a group of returning nurses were asked why they felt they needed a course, they replied:

- 'I don't want to go back apologizing.'
- 'I feel out of touch, rusty, completely incompetent.'
- 'It will be good to be with others doing the same thing.'
- 'I felt secure as a student nurse.'
- 'I feel too vulnerable with drug rounds and dosage.'
- 'All techniques have changed.'
- 'Younger nurses are intolerant of blundering old nurses.'

Most of them added:

- 'I lack confidence to go back.'
- 'The course will give me confidence.'
- 'Although I "catch on" quickly, I don't feel confident enough.'

Any nurse retraining programme therefore needs to contain three main elements:

- A booster to confidence, and reaffirmation of competence.
- A reawakening of appropriate old skills and knowledge.
- A building of new skills and knowledge.

Returning without a course

Many nurses may believe that the reawakening of old skills and knowledge can best be achieved by 'doing it'. This might be a valid assumption up to a point, depending on the skills involved. What might affect the reawakening however will be changes in the equipment and the method as well as the knowledge base which underlies the particular activity. I can best illustrate this with an experience of a nurse who returned to practice:

> 'I had returned to nursing after being out of practice for ten years. I was the only qualified nurse on duty with two auxiliaries on an elderly care ward. I felt that the basic nursing care was poor, so in an attempt to improve it I decided to do a 'back round'. The auxiliary did not know what I meant but willingly joined in the vigorous massaging with soap and water of the buttocks, heels and elbows of the frail elderly patients, followed by the drying and powdering of the same.'

This nurse had had no retraining programme so she could be excused for not knowing about the research which indicates that vigorous massaging of delicate skin tissues can actually destroy them, causing the very sores she was trying to prevent. The new knowledge would have told her that turning the patients at least two-hourly to relieve pressure would have been much more effective. She might have done this coincidentally but not with any application of knowledge.

Unsafe practice

This account demonstrates how awakening of old skills unrelated to changes in the knowledge base might well result in unsafe practice which could be damaging to the patient and demoralizing for the nurse who, when the error is pointed out by colleagues, could suffer a severe dent in confidence.

Another reason for not relying solely on the reawakening of skills and knowledge in the clinical areas is the variable commitment and expertise of the staff themselves. Although all qualified nurses have a professional responsibility to teach their peers and subordinates and a majority of them do discharge this responsibility admirably, it should not be relied on as the only method of updating skills and knowledge, for the following reasons:

(1) Staff are far too often stretched to their limits delivering patient care, with little time or energy to take on the teaching role, particularly with a group who are to all intents and purposes qualified nurses who may be more experienced than the staff themselves.
(2) It is not particularly encouraging and reassuring for a patient to have a qualified nurse learning on-the-job.
(3) There is a danger that teaching will be fragmented, not necessarily following a logical plan or building on previous learning experiences.

(4) The training might be biased, out-of-date and directed at a specific need unrelated to wider issues, e.g. it is quicker to manually lift someone than to use a hoist.
(5) The ward staff might not have acquired teaching skills so will not understand the importance or need of performing this function well, resulting in less than satisfactory learning.
(6) Finally, even a basic orientation is often done skimpily or not at all, leaving the nurses feeling unsure, inadequate and sometimes frightened about the potential problems with which they cannot cope.

Professionally there is a clear obligation for qualified nurses to be accountable for their own practice, which implies that they can state what they are doing, why they are doing it and what the outcome of their actions will be. This requires an up-to-date knowledge and skill base. Furthermore the UKCC states that it is nurses' own responsibility to keep themselves professionally developed to enable them to act as an accountable practitioner.

Changes in practice

A more pragmatic reason for undertaking a Return to Nursing course is the rapid changes that have taken place in the NHS in general and in nursing in particular. Many of these changes are obvious and often well publicized, e.g. no hats, shortage of staff, day surgery and bed closures.

There are many more less obvious changes however which are far more subtle in their influence on nursing practice, e.g. patient allocation as opposed to old style task allocation, and the nursing process which is a systematic approach to care, including assessment, problem identification and the planning of care with the patient.

As one bank nurse found on her first morning back on duty:

'My first experience of this was quite unnerving. I went on to a ward for a morning shift. I was greeted by the ward sister who told me I was to care for three patients, two women and a man. She indicated where they were and walked off. She must have noticed my blank face and sensed my panic because she turned back and added, "Mrs S likes to be 'done' first and the nursing notes are in the trolley by the desk".

I did not know where to start. If the ward sister had told me to help with the breakfasts or the drug round I would have been quite happy as this is what my previous training had taught me to do. Priority setting and decision making, the skills I now required, were not part of my previous learning.'

Another change in practice which many nurses find difficult is the idea of working in collaboration with the patient towards mutually agreed goals, rather than telling the patient what to do. This requires knowledge and skills on the part of the nurse to give patients information to enable them to make choices about their own lifestyle, and to accept their decisions no matter what the nurse thinks should or should not be done.

Anxieties about technology and new equipment always feature highly in returning nurses' identified needs for training. It is true that heart monitoring, intravenous infusions, measured dose infection pumps and continuous bladder irrigations are now commonplace in acute hospitals, but many of these techniques are now finding their way into the community where patients are taught aseptic techniques to care for parenteral nutrition lines, renal dialysis and peritoneal dialysis.

Ward-based laboratory testing, such as blood glucose monitoring, urine testing and tests for occult blood, have become routine and it is expected that qualified nurses are competent in these procedures. But as equipment is continually changing and most nurses can learn to use simple equipment by reading printed instructions, much of the training will occur when and where it is needed.

Success of courses

No course can be all things to all people. The returning nurse is an intelligent, self-directed, highly motivated adult learner who will learn when the stimulus and opportunity is provided. The ability to use a new piece of equipment should not be minimized but by putting the mechanics of nursing in proper perspective the returning nurse begins to see that the ability to meet individual emotional, physical and spiritual needs of patients is still the most important component of good nursing care.

Does a Return to Nursing course meet the needs of the returner? Let the returners themselves have the final say:

- 'The most useful aspect of the course has been regaining confidence in myself as a person but, above that, as a nurse.'
- 'Being able to discuss problems and finding out how the nursing profession has changed and developed.'
- 'Clinical practice was a high spot and it was only then that I felt, Yes this is definitely me!'
- 'Made me more enthusiastic – felt that I definitely have something to offer.'
- 'I feel more updated and have gained satisfactory knowledge to help me in going back to nursing.'

- 'I found being with others who shared many feelings throughout the course very reassuring and confidence building.'
- 'Many topics covered helped to demysticize areas that caused concern.'
- 'At the end of the course I feel very positive about what I have gained. I have re-established what knowledge and skills I have and what I can use to persuade an employer to appoint me.'

Further reading

Books

Lawson, K.H. (1979) *Philosophical Concepts and Values in Adult Education.* Oxford University Press.
Peters, R.S. & Dray, W.H. (1975) *The Philosophy of Education.* Oxford University Press.

Articles

Anon (1980) Government Subsidies. Refresher courses to ease shortages. *RNABC – News,* **12**(6) 4.
Curran, C.L. & Lengacher, C.A. (1982) RN [Registered Nurse] re-entry programmes: programmatic and personal considerations. *Nurse Educator,* **7**(3) 29–32.
Eggland, C.A. (1980) Development and delivery of a refresher course for nurses. *Journal of Continuing Education for Nurses,* **11**(3) 28–43.
King, J. (1973) Come back to nursing – if you dare. *Nursing Times,* **69**(30) 964–5.
Lysaght, L. (1981) Refresher courses for returning nurses. *New Zealand Nurses Journal,* **74**(3) 11–22.
Ruxton, J.P. (1981) Barriers to re-entry: problems are many, solutions few. *California Nurse,* **77**(4) 6.
United Kingdom Central Council (1987) *Exercising Accountability.* UKCC, London.
Watts, M. (1983) The part-timers and evening classes in Portsmouth. *Nursing Times,* **79**(39) 29–30.

Part 3
Back to Practice

Chapter 5
Has Nursing Changed?

Change is an inevitable part of life. Nothing stands still in life or nursing; the status quo is never an option. But change should be an active process which is nurtured and rewarded in order to make it adapt and grow. Individuals will be more ready to change if it is a normal part of the organization's life.

The changes required in nursing will be in the tasks performed, the formal structure in which the work takes place and the informal relations between the people who work there. Anxieties and uncertainties come about when there appears to be little or no control over the degree, pace and direction of the change.

Pace of change

When I returned to nursing in 1977 after thirteen years out of practice I found that very little had changed. I returned to the same Health Authority and after a brief induction period I was able to resume full nursing activities.

About the only two changes I was aware of were the implementation of the 1966 Salmon reorganization of nursing management, and the use of sterile supplies. The first change appeared to be a change in name only from matron, assistant and deputy matron to senior nursing officer and nursing officers respectively. The second change under the name of central sterile supplies department represented a great saving in time and energy. To have all the equipment and dressings supplied already sterilized eliminated the need to boil everything in the sterilizer for twenty minutes before use. Also, the need to pack drums with dressings for autoclaving had been superseded.

However, for the nurses who left nursing in 1977 and are now resuming their careers in the 1990s, is their return so simple or easy? For many, particularly those who return to the non-acute areas of nursing, their immediate impression is that nothing has changed. Basic care remains unchanged; in fact with only qualified nurses around it feels too comfortable. As time passes, however, many subtle changes can emerge which were not always obvious immediately.

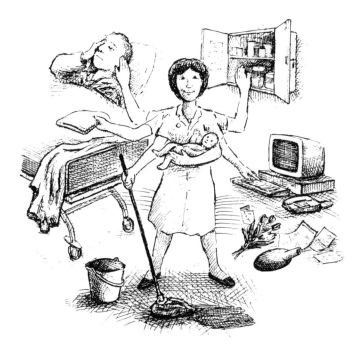

A nurse is a nurse is a nurse is a . . .

Changed attitudes

The returning nurses become aware of changes in the attitudes of the staff and the way care is organized. The work environment is different and the equipment used in that environment is often unfamiliar. The returning nurses realise too that they would have to learn to work within an extended health care team and understand their various roles; also that rapid developments in medicine have 'knock-on' effects on the caring role of the nurse.

Lastly, in recent years there has been a growth in the creation of specialist nurse roles and in specialized nursing, which may challenge returners with their lack of knowledge and rusty skills.

One striking change noted by all returners is the informality between both staff and patients. Using christian names was the most obvious evidence of this, especially with patients. Not all the returners feel comfortable with this change, especially those whose previous experience had been in a fairly rigid, hierarchical system where they would use 'nurse', 'staff' or 'sister' with their colleagues and every patient would have had his or her surname prefixed with their title. Now nurses frequently wear badges showing their christian names.

Calling patients by their first name is not universally liked or accepted by either the patients or nurses. It is interpreted by some as showing a lack of respect, as recounted by a conversation one returner had with an elderly lady:

> 'When I asked the patient what she would like me to call her, she thought for a moment then replied, Mrs X, not Alice, like the cheeky young nurses did, adding that she had not been called Alice since her husband died many years ago.'

Some returners were also surprised that the doctors were called by their christian names, although this usually only applied to the house-men and some senior registrars. This was not too difficult to accept for the older returners as they remarked how young these doctors looked anyway.

Evidence of the informality went beyond the use of christian names. It was demonstrated in the changed attitude of nurses towards the patients and vice versa. Patients were no longer a disease in a bed, waiting to be told what to do and how and when to do it. They were now seen as individuals and partners in care, to be consulted and advised, not dictated to and directed all the time.

More time was spent with the patients, talking with them, giving them choices about how they were going to spend their day and asking them what help they thought they might need. This once again was often difficult for returners to cope with. They were used to a fairly organized system of working, with all the patients bathed or washed and beds made before ten o'clock. Now, horror of horrors, beds remained unmade after lunch and if patients did not want a bath they did not have a bath.

Nurses' attitudes to each other were far more supportive and less critical. They seemed to be aware of the insecurities of the returners and were most kind, helpful and approachable. There seemed far less concern for administrative neatness and convenience and far more concern to help and serve both nurses and patients.

Changes in uniforms

Where have all the hats gone, and even worse, what are nurses wearing as uniform now? Nurses' uniforms have been a debatable issue for a number of years. In the past they were a matter of decoration and distinction and were worn with pride. Their relationship to the work of nurses did not usually enter the debate. Changes in the uniforms have come about gradually over the years, in response to changes in fashion and society and the changes in the daily work of nurses.

The first item affected by these changes was the hat. The elaborate, mainly decorative creation which was a vestige of the nun's habit was slowly replaced by a smaller, though frilly, starched cap. As this remained difficult to maintain for the busy mobile nurse it was abandoned in favour of the obnoxious paper cap.

Although this was easier to maintain and carry about, and of course was much cheaper, it served no useful purpose at all. It neither covered the head to give protection nor adorned the wearer. It was easily knocked off when, for instance, nurses needed to get close to patient to lift them. Worse still, it was discovered that the paper cap, which was usually left around made up for weeks, collected dust and bacteria from the atmosphere which was then deposited by the nurse every time she bent forward.

Although some Health Authorities and some nurses still prefer to retain the cap, many are now accustomed to a nurse being without a cap.

Most returning female nurses can now accept and understand why caps have been abandoned, but very few can condone a rejection of the uniform dress. Uniform dresses have changed considerably over the years: the hemline has gone up and down as fashion dictated; the starched apron, collar and cuffs were discarded in the late 1950s as disposable plastic aprons were introduced; and there were attempts in the 1970s to introduce a national uniform of blue and white check. This was taken up by some Health Authorities but many preferred to retain their traditional colours and styles.

There has been some attempt to make dresses more roomy to allow the nurse freedom of movement, particularly when lifting or handling patients. What has never been accepted by female nurses generally is the introduction of trousers or culottes. Even though they would be much better suited to the physical activities of nursing, and would be safer in that they would give the wearer more freedom to move, very few nurses wear them.

So far only two nursing specialities have completely abandoned uniform: learning disabilities and psychiatry. It was felt by many that the uniform actually created a barrier between the nurse and patient and prevented nurses establishing a therapeutic relationship with their patients.

Some areas in general nursing are now experimenting with wearing their own clothes rather than uniform, but this experiment has been resisted by both staff and patients. Staff are worried about transferring infection from hospital to home and vice versa. Patients' worries centre around the inability to identify individuals in the health care team.

This worry was reflected in the experiences of returners, as they initially went on to the wards with tabards over their own clothes. One was at the nursing station when a physiotherapist asked for help. When the returner stepped forward the physiotherapist said she did not want a relative, she wanted a nurse. The returners have also been mistaken for domestic staff and spent an inordinate amount of time explaining who they were and what they were doing.

There is of course a big risk in putting returners in trained nurses' uniforms: the expectations of everyone with whom they come into contact will be more than most of them can cope with initially.

Uniforms serve two main purposes: as protective clothing and for easy identification. Those areas where uniform has been discarded have not suffered unduly, either from infection or lack of identification. It is interesting that in those areas the nurses seem to have adopted an informal uniform of either jeans and T-shirts or dark coloured track suits; and most wear a large, clearly-displayed, name badge to aid identification.

Changes in wards

The fact that the actual ward environment had changed architecturally seemed to bother only a few returning nurses. Certainly most of the modern general hospitals are designed with wards of small, four or six-bedded bays, with a nursing station strategically placed somewhere in the middle. Nobody seemed to miss the large Florence Nightingale type wards where everyone could see what everyone else was doing. A few nurses complained about the fact that they spent a good deal of time walking around while caring for patients in different bays.

Some nurses were disappointed to find that the sluice had disappeared, replaced by the dirty utility room, a title which did not have the same ring to it. For most the layout of the ward and finding out where everything was kept was fairly easy.

What most found disturbing were the empty beds and shortage of staff, something unheard of only a few years ago. Another source of concern was the untidy, dirty state of some of the wards. For many returners these represented a lowering of standards from those to which they had been accustomed in the past. One welcome addition in many areas was the provision of a resources room for the staff.

Changes in equipment and systems

As already mentioned in earlier chapters, equipment is constantly changing. As new ways of working are introduced and there are new developments in the diagnosing and treatment of patients, equipment has to change and adapt to accommodate new practice. Returning nurses are not only daunted by new, highly technical equipment but can be easily 'thrown' by changes in familiar everyday equipment such as drug trolleys, dressing packs and beds.

Drugs

The first drug round nurses undertake after returning to practice can be a very worrying experience and many have admitted it has taken them several hours to complete. The drug trolley itself varies; it can range from the standard trolley with stock bottles which lock into their own space, to a compartmentalized trolley with a drawer for each patient. In some areas patients have their own locked compartment in their bedside locker. Drug charts are also a worry, with illegible writing, unfamiliar abbreviations and the drug names differing from chart to bottle.

Another change is the identification of the patient. Name bands are not always worn or they may become obliterated or are removed when the patient receives treatment. Sometimes photographs are included on the drug chart, which can help with identification providing they are kept up-to-date. Other unfamiliar equipment encountered by returning nurses includes syringe pumps, drip monitors and continuous infusion of drugs such as morphine.

Dressings

The familiar task of 'doing a dressing' can trip up many an unwary nurse. The use of Central Sterile Supplies can make life so much easier, but the packets do not always indicate the contents. In addition, the equipment contained within them may not always be easy to handle, e.g. plastic forceps can be slippery and have a tendency to cross over when attempting to grip an object.

Dressings, sutures and clips may have changed too, and the method of suturing could well be different. The need to suture in a more cosmetic way, reducing ugly scarring, has meant the use of continuous and subcutaneous sutures with beads either end to identify them, for ease of removal.

The whole management of wounds, whether they are clean surgical wounds or deep ulcers, has changed over the past five to ten years. The use of occlusive dressings, such as op-site, which can remain in place for several days, eliminates the need for daily or twice daily dressing rounds.

Disposal systems

Disposal of equipment is more carefully organized now. Sharps disposal continues to be a source of debate and the equipment to achieve this varies considerably between Health Authorities. The Department of Health has laid down that needles should not be covered before disposal but should be placed directly into a suitable container. Some containers are made of rigid plastic, but others are made of cardboard which can be pierced by the unguarded needle causing damage to whoever picks up the box.

Instruments used in aseptic procedures can usually be sent for sterilization and re-use. A separate bag is provided for this purpose. Disposal of rubbish is now colour coded and waste must be placed in the correct coloured bag or it might end up in the wrong disposal system.

Beds

The humble hospital bed should not cause any problems, yet many nurses have wrestled with adjusting the height, getting cot sides down, and finding a bed stripper. There are many, new, quite sophisticated designs of bed now on the market which can turn the patient at the push of a button, relieve pressure in preselected areas, or suspend the patient above the mattress in a net. In some areas with certain categories of patients, top bed clothes have been replaced with duvets which are more comfortable for the patient and cut down considerably on bed-making. Another welcome addition to the bed is the use of in-continence sheets which ensure the patient no longer lies in a wet bed.

Interesting additions to some wards, particularly long stay wards, are washing machines, clothes dryers and even in one case a jacuzzi. This of course meant thas someone has to be employed to use this machinery but it does help to retain patients' own clothes.

Aromatherapy

A very pleasant change noted by some returners was the smell of the wards. Aromatherapy and massage with essential oils are becoming much more common in a whole range of wards. This means that the perfumes used pervade not only the rooms in which they are used but sometimes the whole ward. This is very welcome, particularly in wards where the smell of stale urine and worse commonly greeted you as you opened the ward door.

Changes in staffing

One change noted by nurses when they returned was the developing concept of being part of a team delivering care for the patient. Where this was well developed it was recognized that each member of the team had an important contribution to make. It was also recognized that as nurses provided continuity of care over 24 hours, they were usually the ones who co-ordinated the care. It is much more common now for the team to have case conferences where all interested parties are involved. These might include the physiotherapist, occupational therapist, dietician, medical social worker, nurse and doctor. The patient and/or relatives might also be included, if this is appropriate.

Also, when nurses plan care they consult with and ask advice from any member of the team who has the knowledge and expertise. For many returners this idea of collaboration was far removed from their previous experience of other members of the team visiting the patient to 'do their bit', and going away often without even talking to the nursing staff.

Services contracted out

The contracting out of hospital services, such as catering, cleaning and supplies departments, has meant a major rethink for nursing staff. They may not have their own domestic staff with whom they can build a relationship and have some control over the work they do and the standard they achieve. Disputes over how the ward is cleaned and whose responsibility it is to mop up after patients and staff, are more likely to be settled with the supervisor than with the domestic concerned. What is written in the contract and who determines this becomes quite critical.

Serving meals

In some areas distributing food to patients has become a non-nursing job, though feeding patients and recording fluid intake remains the responsibility of the nurse. Many returning nurses regret the loss of the social occasion of meal times when patients were served an appropriate meal from a heated trolley in the middle of the ward and a careful check was kept on how much each individual ate.

Contracts for supplies

Contracts for supplying goods to hospitals and wards are keenly competed for, with the user often having little or no say in the matter. This means that as contracts are awarded for fixed periods of time, unless the contractor remains competitive he could well lose the contract next time round. Although financially this may be applauded, from a practical point of view it can be very confusing for nursing staff if fairly basic equipment changes, as noted by two returners:

'I was asked to empty a urinary drainage bag, something I had done on previous occasions successfully. I placed a receiver under the outlet and turned the knob. Nothing happened. I twisted it the other way still no luck. I felt so stupid I did not want to ask how to empty the bag, so I fiddled with it until suddenly my hands were washed in the escaping urine. I discovered afterwards that the contract for urinary drainage systems had changed and I should have pushed the tap across.'

'The intravenous infusion bag of my patient was just about empty so I collected a new bag to replace it. I unsealed what I thought was the inlet channel and tried to insert the giving set. It just would not go in. After several unsuccessful attempts I called a colleague for help. I had been using the wrong opening; it was of course easy when I used the correct one. It was then I discovered that the contract for intraveous fluids had changed, and the arrangement of portholes for giving sets was very different.'

With so much equipment in use and so many changes occurring it is very difficult for even the permanent staff to be competent all the time.

Patient turnover

Unless a returning nurse works on a long stay, elderly care ward, or maybe in psychiatry, she cannot fail to notice the rapid turnover of patients. The average stay for patients in acute general hospitals is between four and five days. This means that if a nurse works only once a week she will probably have to get to know a whole ward of new patients each time she works. It also implies that most of the patients on the ward will be quite dependent, needing a great deal of nursing care.

On an acute surgical ward the nurse might be involved in preparation and planning care pre-operatively. She will also give post-operative care, at least for the first 24 hours. Most patients will be mobilized in this time and probably will be given pain relief. As indicated earlier, wounds will only be redressed if required. As soon as drips and drains are removed and patients are able to walk, they will quite likely be discharged either to a local community or cottage hospital or even home if this is possible. Their care will then be supervised by their own general practitioner who will arrange for clips or sutures to be removed.

Medical patients too will not occupy an acute hospital bed for longer than it takes to diagnose disease and prescribe care. The prescription will be carried out either at home or in a community hospital. Nurses often become involved in trying to prevent the premature discharge of patients which can result in re-admission within the next 24 to 36 hours.

Medical advances

Other more recent medical advances have profoundly changed the nursing care required by the patients. Innovations include:

- Micro surgery, particularly in abdominal and orthopaedic operations; for example appendectomy and meniscectomy.
- Less traumatic surgery for breast cancers and gynaecological operations such as hysterectomy.
- Non-invasive techniques using laser beams for crushing and dispersing gall bladder and kidney stones, and quite recently for shrinking prostate glands.

All the above require only minimal stay in hospital and minimal pre- and post-operative care. Diagnostic techniques have also improved, making diagnosis more accurate and less traumatic. The use of endoscopy for bowel and stomach problems can incorporate examination and treatment without the need for general anaesthetic. Whole body scanning can accurately pinpoint trouble spots and act as a definitive guide for treatment.

Almost all of these techniques can be performed as day cases, eliminating the need for hospitalization. Most hospitals now have day wards to cater for patients who can come into hospital prepared, receive treatment and go home the same day. These wards are often open 9 AM to 5 AM Monday to Friday, which suits many returners who can only offer limited times for work while their children are at school. There are drawbacks in that the work is limited in scope and can become boring and repetitious, with little challenge or stimulation.

Specialized nursing

A very gradual change over the past 30 years or so has been the emergence of specialized nursing and specialist nurses. It is inevitable that as doctors develop knowledge and expertise in the treatment of disease, they will set up specialist units for that purpose. These units will also require nurses to care for the patients. It is just as inevitable therefore that nurses will develop knowledge and expertise in the care of patients suffering from particular diseases.

These specialist units range from the highly technical Intensive Care Units or premature baby units to specialist surgical units such as heart and kidney transplant, stroke rehabilitation units, and the hospice palliative care units. The prospect of working in the highly technical areas, such as intensive care or transplant or dialysis wards, frightens most returning nurses. Many however feel quite able to cope with the demands of rehabilitation and hospice care wards.

Apart from the nurse who becomes an expert in a certain field of nursing, such as medicine or surgery, there is a growing trend for nurses to set themselves up as specialists in a range of nursing activities. These will include stoma therapy, infection control, parenteral nutrition, incontinence advice and AIDS counselling, to name but a few.

A great deal of knowledge and expertise will be invested in these individuals, which can only benefit the patient. The danger lies in the fact that the rest of the nurses hand over all responsibility in the specialized area of nursing, and subsequently become de-skilled. The sensible way to use the specialist nurse is in the same way as the nurse would use the skills and knowledge of other members of the health care team: for help and advice.

Of course, not all the changes mentioned in this chapter will be experienced by all nurses returning to work. Equally, there are bound to be other changes not mentioned here, as nothing stands still. It is important that changes are not seen as a deterrent to returners but rather as a stimulation or motivation, as stated by one returner:

'Hooray! Nurses are now encouraged to question, think for themselves, evaluate, be assertive, actively take their lives in their own hands, articulate, and use their common sense, experience and intelligence.'

Further reading

Books

Broome, A. (1990) *Managing Change*. Macmillan, London.

Dean, D.J. (1987) *Manpower Solutions*. RCN/Scutari Press, London.

Mackay, L. (1989) *Nursing a Problem*. Open University Press, Milton Keynes.

Snowball, J. & Green, W. (1987) *Nursing Principles*, 2nd edn. Blackwell Scientific Publications, Oxford.

United Kingdom Central Council (1986) *Advisory Document: Administration of Medicines*. UKCC, London.

United Kingdom Central Council (1992) *Code of Professional Conduct*. UKCC, London.

Articles

Dixon, M. (1988) Back to nursing – a sham. *Professional Nurse*, **3**(4) 119.

Murray, S. (1978) Back to nursing. *Nursing Times*, **74**(22) 904–905.

Schrock, R.A. (1977) On political consciousness in nurses. *Journal of Advanced Nursing*, **2** 41–50.

Chapter 6
Professional Practice, Knowledge and Skills

The speed with which new knowledge and changes in practice are developing in nursing creates difficulties for the returning nurse searching for meaning from an avalanche of nursing books and journals. In addition, nursing practice today includes a much broader range of activities than that represented by the traditional image of the nurse at the bedside of the sick patient. This expanding role, which is constantly changing in response to societal needs, requires appropriate knowledge and competence in practical skills.

This chapter describes and reflects on the changes and trends that have an effect on nursing practice, both from a national and international perspective. The focus is on the fundamentals of nursing care to enable nurses to identify their own nursing values. The need to study further to give confidence to practise in and understand the modern world of nursing, is also emphasized.

Changes in how nursing is perceived and practised in this country over the past decade have been influenced by the deliberations and actions of such bodies as the United Kingdom Central Council, European Community, World Health Organization, International Council of Nurses, the National Health Service Executive and various political groups.

Code of conduct

The United Kingdom Central Council was established by an Act of Parliament, the Nurses, Midwives and Health Visitors Act 1979, to replace the various bodies which were responsible for nursing, midwifery and health visiting, such as the General Nursing Council. One of the first actions of the UKCC was to write a Code of Professional Conduct.

This code forms a keystone for professional nursing practice in the UK. Although not a legal document in itself it will be referred to by the Professional Conduct Committee when considering a case of professional misconduct, so it in effect sets the standard by which professional nursing is practised.

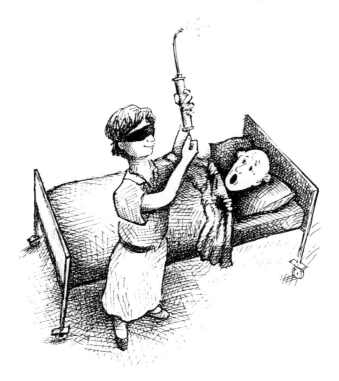

Practice without knowledge is blind.

The Code is based on the issue of accountability, mentioned in Chapter 4. Unless nurses are accountable for their own practice they cannot act in a professional way. Furthermore the code indicates that registered practitioners are accountable for their actions as professionals at all times, whether engaged in current practice or not and whether on or off duty, as stated in the UKCC advisory document *Exercising Accountability.*

The document argues further that accountability must be an integral part of professional practice, since, in the course of that practice, the practitioner has to make judgements in a wide variety of circumstances and be answerable for those judgements. The document does not set out the variety of circumstance but instead describes the basic principles which underlie the exercise of accountability, summarized in the document as follows:

(1) The interests of the patient or client are paramount.
(2) Professional accountability must be exercised in such a manner as to ensure that the primacy of the interests of patients or clients is

respected and must not be overridden by those of the professions or their practitioners.

(3) The exercise of accountability requires the practitioner to seek to achieve and maintain high standards.

(4) Advocacy on behalf of patients or clients is an essential feature of the exercise of accountability by a professional practitioner.

(5) The role of other persons in the delivery of health care to patients or clients must be recognized and respected, provided that the first principle above is honoured.

(6) Public trust and confidence in the profession are dependent on its practitioners being seen to exercise their accountability responsibly.

(7) Each registered nurse, midwife or health visitor must be able to justify any action or decision not to act taken in the course of professional practice.

Organization of care

This document leaves no doubt about the person to whom the professional is accountable or who is the focus of nursing care: the patient or client. This implies that care is organized in such a way that it is the patient rather than the task which is important.

For many nurses who trained in the past, and even some today, who have nursed using a task allocation system, it is difficult to put the interests of the patient first; for example, a common practice even today is to have every patient bathed before 10 AM. The practitioner never asks why this is done, whether it is necessary or even more important whether it is in the best interest of the patient. It can be argued that for some patients a bath in the morning is necessary, if for instance they have had a sticky, uncomfortable night, if they are going for surgery or investigation that day or if they have been incontinent. But it might be more difficult to justify such an action on routine grounds for all patients, whether they feel they need a bath or not.

Another reason put forward for bathing patients before 10 AM was to have them ready for the doctor's round, or to have completed the baths before the ward was cleaned. Neither reason really puts the interest of patients first or respects their right to decide if and when they should bathe.

Accountability for one's actions

For many nurses, but particularly returning nurses, the idea of being accountable for one's own practice is quite alarming at first. To take responsibility for your actions, to question what you have done, how you have accomplished it and whether the decisions taken were right or wrong is quite alien to many returning nurses. They were used to 'obeying orders', 'doing what they were told' and 'hiding behind Sister's skirts' when things went wrong. They might seriously question whether they are free or willing to accept accountability for their own decision making, and would prefer an upward delegation of that responsibility. This is usually only an initial reaction to a new concept which given time becomes acceptable, as stated by one returning nurse at the end of the course:

> 'Basic nursing care is no different but now nurses know why they are doing what they are doing.'

However, nurses are not only accountable for what they do but must also accept accountability for what they do not do in the course of professional practice. This was well illustrated by one returning nurse who came back to class very distressed by what she saw as low standards of care after an evening shift on an elderly care ward:

> 'There were 18 patients on the ward, only three of whom could get out of bed. An experienced enrolled nurse was in charge, with an auxiliary nurse to help her. She was unable to get any relief from the general office. She decided that after supper the most important thing was to turn and toilet the patients, changing bed linen as needed. They could not be given their usual warm milky drink but they would have water or squash when they were turned.'

The returning nurse thought this was an appalling decision and the patients should have been given their milky drinks; but she could not explain how this could be achieved in the circumstances. The enrolled nurse documented the incident explaining the decision she had taken and why, including the fact that the patients were denied their normal bedtime drink.

Decisions about nursing care are not always easy but one returning nurse was comforted by the fact that it was quite permissible, indeed expected, that she would refuse to undertake any work if she was unsure or untrained to do it. It is recognized that the prerequisites for accepting accountability for decisions must be:

- An ability to undertake the work.
- Knowledge on which to base decisions about the work.
- Skills which may be needed to competently carry out the work.
- A value system or beliefs about nursing which will guide practice.

Beliefs about nursing

What individual nurses believe about nursing will depend on a number of factors, ranging from their own cultural and educational background and where and when they trained, to their experiences of life. 'This set of beliefs is often so much an innate part of the personality, unexpressed and maybe unexpressible, that it forms a blueprint or model of nursing around which practice is shaped.

When required, most nurses can express their beliefs in a few sentences; for example:

'We believe that the patient is a unique individual with physical, spiritual, social and emotional needs. The patient is the centre of our entire nursing focus and has the right to considerate, honest and respectful care. He/she has the right to privacy in all aspects of that care. The patient is part of a family unit and when appropriate and feasible, the family is included in the planning, implementation and education process.

'We believe that nursing is a dynamic profession which demands a strong sense of responsibility and commitment from the individual. The nurse accepts a personal responsibility to remain current with modern trends within the profession. The nursing process of assessment planning, intervention and evaluation is a critical component of nursing care. A quality assurance programme within nursing is essential in order to identify patient and staff needs. The professional nurse has a direct responsibility to train peers and subordinates.

'We believe that the hospital is basically an organization of those individuals who constitute the health care team. These people are representative of professions and organizations and perform specialized work in which all of their skills and achievements are focused on the primary goal of patient care. This service has the responsibility of maintaining good lines of communication and giving appropriate support to these individuals and services.'

Not all nurses will necessarily agree with all the above statements. This does not imply that anyone is wrong or right but suggests that we do need to be honest and acknowledge our beliefs so that we can understand from whence our nursing practice is derived.

If, for example, you believe that work is the most important thing and that you are there to get a job completed to the best of your ability, this might well conflict with the best interests of the patient. You might therefore be very uncomfortable in a work situation where it was not considered important to have all the baths completed by 10 AM.

Model of care

Our beliefs give us all a model of practice that forms the framework around which we plan our care. The model might be to meet the daily

living needs of the patients which they are unable to meet for themselves, or to help the patients towards self care, or to maintain balance
or equilibrium between needs and deficiencies. The model will depend
not only on our beliefs but also on the kind of patients we are caring
for and the circumstances in which care is delivered.

Whatever model of nursing we adopt, a systematic problem-oriented
approach to planning nursing care is needed. This approach to
decision-making and planning is commonly called the nursing process
and was adopted by the GNC in 1977.

This, like any other process, requires a scientific basis for planning,
decision-making and evaluating outcomes effectively. It is recognized
that certain, common stages have to be achieved for the desired
outcome to be accomplished. The name and number of stages may
vary depending on the nurse and their sources of education. The basic
principles however remain the same.

The nursing process

The four stages of the nursing process may be identified as assessment,
planning, implementation and evaluation. These should not however
be thought of as steps going up, but rather as cyclical with each stage
inter-related with a need for reassessment and modification of plans as
evaluation occurs.

Assessment

The initial stage to any decision making or problem solving must be an
assessment of the situation to gather information on which decisions
can be based. So when nurses first come into contact with a patient or
client they will gather data or facts about the patient. What information,
how much and how soon this is collected will vary depending on the
patient, the circumstances and what information is required. There are
usually three broad headings under which the information is gathered:

(1) Biographical detail such as name, date of birth, address, marital
    status.
(2) Medical information such as diagnosis, reason for admission,
    previous medical history, drugs and allergies.
(3) Personal facts often related to daily activities of living such as
    eating, sleeping, eliminating and mobility – what the normal state is
    and what the present status is with regard to these activities.

This information is usually recorded on a pre-printed form with which
most nurses are familiar. Biographical and medical information has
always been recorded, but the personal facts will be new to many

nurses. The type and amount of information recorded about the personal details of patients will depend on the model of nursing being used. A checklist for collecting this information might be the 14 activities of daily living as identified by Roper, Logan & Tierney in *The Elements of Nursing* (1985) (see Further Reading). These are recognized as the normal activities engaged in by the adult to maintain independent living:

(1) Breathe normally.
(2) Eat and drink adequately.
(3) Eliminate body wastes.
(4) Move and maintain desirable postures.
(5) Sleep and rest.
(6) Select suitable clothes, dress and undress.
(7) Maintain body temperature within normal range by adjusting clothing and modifying the environment.
(8) Keep the body clean and well groomed and protect the integument.
(9) Avoid danger in the environment and avoid injuring others.
(10) Communicate with others in expressing emotions, needs, fears or opinions.
(11) Worship according to one's faith.
(12) Work in such a way that there is a sense of accomplishment.
(13) Play or participate in various forms of recreation.
(14) Learn, discover or satisfy the curiosity that leads to normal development and health and use the available health facilities.

Nursing history of the patient
The nursing history of the patient will not necessarily be taken on admission of the patient but may be collected over the first 48 hours following admission. Sources used may be the old medical records if there have been previous admissions, current records already obtained from other departments such as outpatients or emergency admissions, the patient and relatives and friends of the patient, and other members of the health care team who have been asked to assess the patient. The subsequent plan of care for the patient will only be as good as the information collected on the history of the patient. Time and skill spent over data gathering will be evident in the next stages of the process.

Many returning nurses will argue that they have always taken a nursing history of their patients but an investigation of past nursing records shows that this was not always accomplished in a systematic way nor in sufficient detail to either identify problems, set goals or plan carefully. It is only in recent years that nurses have developed the skills needed for data collection. The skills include interviewing and communication with people, and observation in both a subjective way and more objective measurement. These cannot be explored in depth but it is worth mentioning here that most returning nurses have, as noted in Chapter 2, well developed communication and observation skills.

Identifying problems
Having gathered all the information about the patient which is felt necessary and appropriate, the next stage is to review the information so as to identify problems the patient has with daily living activities, which will require nursing intervention. For many returning nurses this will be an aspect of care for which they have had little previous experience. To identify problems we need to know and understand normal functioning and compare this with the normal functioning of the individual and how it has been compromised by the patient's current condition. To do this a knowledge of anatomical, physiological, psychological and social functioning is required.

Identification of problems should be carried out *with* the patient if at all possible and should not be done *to* the patient. In identifying a problem the nurse is making a clinical judgement about the actual or potential response of an individual to given health problems. It should be expressed in a concise statement which describes the problem and its aetiology if known. This will then indicate the nursing intervention required for which the nurse is accountable.

For example, a patient might have a problem walking. This could be for a number of reasons so the nurse will know from her assessment which is the most likely reason, e.g. painful arthritic knees. It could have been related to a broken leg, old age, paralysis, amputation or a fear of falling. Knowing the reason will indicate the care needed.

After assessing the patient it should be possible to draw up a list of problems the patient describes, plus potential problems that might develop if preventive action is not taken. A further refinement of the list of problems would be to prioritize them, putting those requiring immediate action first.

Goal setting
It should now be possible to draw up a plan of care based on the list of identified problems. Some nurses like to set goals or outcomes for each problem. This is useful when evaluating care, to measure whether the goal has been reached. There are nurses who feel this is an intellectual exercise and would argue that the goal is built into the plan of care. Others however, at least initially, find that writing out goals with the patient gives them both a sense of achievement when goals are successfully accomplished. If they are not accomplished, then there is a clear indication that the plan of care is not working for some reason.

If a goal is to be written down it is important that it is clear, concise and unambiguous and agreed with the patient if possible. For example, the patient who has a problem walking due to painful arthritic knees could expect to walk with minimal pain within 24 hours of admission. The nurse would need more information than supplied above to determine such a goal. If the patient has suffered arthritis in the knees for a number of years the joint capsule is likely to be badly damaged and it might be difficult without a great deal of intensive treatment to reduce pain when walking. The goal therefore needs also to be realistic and achievable. This once again demands knowledge and some expertise from the nurse who is determining the goal.

Most returning nurses, unless they have managed to maintain their knowledge level in particular areas of clinical speciality, will need time before they feel competent to undertake this aspect of care.

Care planning

The next stage in the process is devising a plan of care for each of the identified problems. This once again needs to be a concise statement of nursing actions to achieve the desired outcomes and should include how these may be achieved and, if appropriate, how frequently. For example, for the aforementioned patient with difficulty walking:

- 'Prescribed analgesia given regularly.'
- 'Pain chart recorded by patient after walking.'
- 'Appropriate walking aid such as a frame made available for patient to assist walking.'

Prescribing effective nursing actions for an identified patient problem is the centre of professional nursing practice. The action must be directed at the individual patient problem and must be grounded in a sound rationale which if possible has been research based. Otherwise the action could be dangerous or a waste of time, e.g. the returning nurse in Chapter 4 deciding to do a 'back round'. This was not meeting any individual problem and was based on knowledge which had been superseded by research which proved the practice dangerous.

Knowledge base

If the nursing action is to be effective, once again the nurse must have a sound knowledge base. It requires a knowledge not only of the effect the disease may have on the daily living activities, but also of the alternative forms of nursing actions. It also requires the ability to select the action best suited to patients' problems, their aetiology and pathology.

There are very few returning nurses who would feel confident enough in their knowledge base to undertake this aspect of care immediately. Given time and resources however most will be able to design a care plan under more expert supervision. There are many nursing books and journals available now which are written specifically around a process format of care, using a nursing model. Very few nursing books are now written using a medical model of disease, pathology, diagnosis, prognosis and medical treatment.

Implementation of care

The proof of any written plan must be in its implementation. As nursing care must cover a 24 hour period it follows that the person writing the plan will not necessarily be the person who has to implement it. The need for good written communication is therefore essential. For any plan to be implemented effectively it is also essential that the right environment is provided and adequate resources are identified both human and material. It is no use for instance stating the patient needs a frame for walking if there are no suitable frames available, or putting a patient who needs the toilet frequently in a bed furthest away from the toilet.

A cause of much frustration and dissatisfaction in nursing today is caused by a mismatch of prescribed nursing care and resources to deliver that care, such as not enough staff of the right calibre, or not enough or worse still no equipment to do the job. The UKCC Code of Professional Conduct (3rd edition, June 1992) quite clearly states that each nurse must:

'12. Report to an appropriate person or authority any circumstances in which safe and appropriate care for patients and clients cannot be provided.'

How care is organized and who implements it will be the responsibility of the ward or department manager. A variety of titles are used, from the more familiar ward sister or charge nurse to senior nurse, co-ordinator or lecturer practitioner. Nursing care may be organized in three main ways: task allocation, team nursing or primary nursing. Sometimes there will be a mixture of two of these and occasionally there will be a reversion back to another system, usually because of inadequate staffing or resources.

Task allocation
Task allocation has already been mentioned. The usual description is that nurses are allocated tasks to do for all or a group of patients, e.g.

the temperatures or washes or drugs. This is an efficient method for ensuring the work is done but it seldoms allows a patient to identify an individual nurse who is responsible for their care.

This is not to say that the nurses are not conscientious and careful in their work or that the work is allocated inappropriately; it is just that it is more difficult to see the patient as a whole individual and more than just the sum of the parts, if you are only dealing with the parts. Physical care may be well attended to but by a number of different people over a 24 hour period. Patients will find it difficult to identify with an individual nurse and so fail to share any fears or anxieties they may have either about their condition or their social circumstances. Patients may be reluctant to take the time of what they see as a busy nurse.

One nurse recalled an incident with an elderly man whom she was sent to assist when he took his daily bath. The patient had been in hospital for many weeks following a severe stroke. He was paralysed down his left side and had difficulty with his speech. As the nurse collected together his toilet requisites the patient showed obvious signs of distress. The nurse drew the curtains round the bed and sat down to devote time to finding out the problem.

With great difficulty the patient told her that the previous day he had been taken to the home to which he was being discharged. Although it was a pleasant home and they had made him very welcome he did not want to go there; he wanted to go to his own flat. 'They' had decided he could not manage there in his present condition and had made alternative arrangements, it seemed, without consulting him. The staff all thought he was happy going to the home; no one had understood how he felt. Fortunately the nurse managed to get the discharge stopped and a rehabilitation programme instituted instead.

Team nursing
An alternative to task allocation may be team nursing. A team of nurses, usually comprising a qualified nurse and maybe a student nurse and an auxiliary, will give care to a group of patients. These may be in a geographical location, e.g. one half of the ward, or may be scattered to give a range of dependency. Sometimes the patients are allocated to individuals in the team who are responsible for giving care prescribed by the team leader, or alternatively individuals will be responsible for tasks for all the patients in the group.

Primary nursing
The third system, primary nursing, is when a qualified, experienced nurse is responsible for the complete care of an individual patient from admission to discharge. The nurse will assess the patient, determine their needs, prescribe care and deliver the care when on duty. An

associate nurse will deliver the care when the primary nurse is off duty, usually following the plan of care prescribed by the primary nurse.

Evaluation of care

The final stage in the process is evaluation; that is, determining whether the care given has met the needs of the patient. This is easier to measure if goals or outcomes have been clearly stated, e.g. for the patient who had a problem walking due to painful arthritic knees, a goal was set to have her walking with minimal pain within 24 hours. The patient would then have been reviewed after 24 hours to determine whether she still had a problem walking. If the problem no longer existed it could be said the plan of care had been successful and so long as it was in operation the patient would be able to walk.

However in the real world problems are never solved that easily and the care might well have to be adjusted after reassessment of the problem. This demonstrates the dynamic nature of the nursing process where care may need to be frequently readjusted as the patient's circumstances change.

Advantages of the nursing process

There has been much criticism of the nursing process over the years, both from within the profession itself and from other members of the health care team. Most of the criticism centres around the amount of time it takes and the increase in paperwork which requires more staff. Patients have also complained about the repetition of the questions and sometimes the irrelevance, like asking men their menstrual history.

Some patients object to being partners in their care and prefer to have someone else do everything for them. However, used correctly as a tool it can only enhance nursing care for several easily identified reasons:

(1) Care has to be individualized and patient focused.
(2) Care is much more likely to be continuous and not dependent on interpretation by different nurses.
(3) Care is not dependent on an individual's memory, thus avoiding care being omitted or forgotten, especially when the nurses are under pressure.
(4) There is less danger of information being heard incorrectly or not at all.

Success in the use of the nursing process depends on the nurse having the confidence and competence to implement it effectively. Nurses must be aware of their responsibility for, and be involved in, making appropriate decisions in diverse environments and circumstances.

Being irresponsible when choosing or using a method of nursing can be just as damaging to patients as any other poor practice. An example of this was given by a returning nurse on a paediatric ward:

> 'A nine-month-old baby suffering from hydrocephalus had been abandoned by his parents when they were informed that he had a poor prognosis. The baby was given extra fuss and attention from all the nurses and continued to thrive in spite of its prognosis. It was decided that the time had come to wean the baby off the bottle. No rational decision was given either for the delayed weaning or why the baby should be weaned at this time. Neither was any plan for weaning drawn up. Consequently each nurse introduced solid food according to her own preference. The result was that after two days the baby suffered severe diarrhoea and attempts to wean were abandoned.'

This demonstrates that practice without knowledge is blind. Nurses can no longer avoid the need to maintain and improve their professional knowledge and competence.

Further reading

Books

Dugas, B.W. (1977) *Introduction to Patient Care.* W.B. Saunders & Co, Philadelphia.

Hunt, P. & Sendell, B. (1983) *Nursing the Adult with a Specific Physiological Disturbance.* Macmillan Education Ltd, London.

McFarlane & Castledine (1983) *The Practice of Nursing.* C.V. Mosby & Co, London.

Roper, N., Logan, W.W. & Tierney, A.J. (1985) *The Elements of Nursing*, 2nd edn. Churchill Livingstone, Edinburgh.

Snowball, J. & Green, W. (1987) *Nursing Principles*, 2nd edn. Blackwell Scientific Publications, Oxford.

United Kingdom Central Council (1989) *Advisory Document: Exercising Accountability.* UKCC, London.

United Kingdom Central Council (1992) *Code of Professional Conduct.* UKCC, London.

Articles

Davies, E. (1983) Does money make a difference? *Nursing Times,* **79**(39) 35–6.

Jackson, A. (1983) The practitioner's view. *Nursing Times,* **79**(36) 67–8.

Pyne, R. (1983) Grasping the legal nettle. *Nursing Times,* **79**(39) 36–8.

Rhodes, B. (1983) Alternative perspectives. *Nursing Times,* **79**(36) 65–6.

Chapter 7
Practical Experience

Starting any new job can be a daunting experience for most people. Although there may well be feelings of excitement and anticipation, these could be countered by fear of the unknown and doubts about one's ability to cope. It can take a great deal of courage to physically open the door and walk into a new working situation. As most of the people there will be strangers to you, and you to them, there is an impression of all eyes focusing on you and everyone watching all that you do and say.

Nursing is particularly threatening in this respect, especially if the nurse is already qualified and thinks, however erroneously, that she should know it all. As one returner explained:

'I used to feel in control both practically and medically but I realize that technology has really revolutionized nursing and the knowlege of drugs has intensified greatly.'

As discussed in Chapter 1, many nurses who have been out of practice for a number of years recollect nursing as a submissive, subordinate, obedient role to an authoritarian figure. Nurses' actions were largely determined by procedures and policies laid down by the bureaucratic institution, and of course by following doctors' orders. The very act of donning a uniform and cap and tying the laces of the regulation black or brown low-heeled shoes is symbolic of donning 'the role' of the nurse, as described by one returner:

'When I return to nursing and put my uniform on there are going to be things I am unsure about, and you are expected to know what you are doing. I am sure once I start it will all fall into place and I will wonder what I was worrying about.'

Preparation for the return

Preparation for the clinical placement and a well planned orientation are considered essential prerequisites for the returning nurse. As one returner explained:

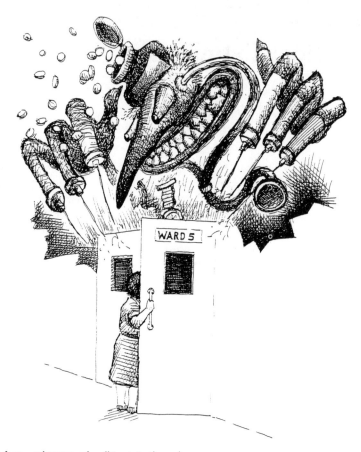

The fears and terrors of walking into the unknown.

'The time spent on the clinical area was made valuable by the time spent preparing for the experience, which much reduced anxieties, and then the sharing of experience.'

The knowledge base has already been discussed in Chapter 6. In addition to the knowledge base, an introduction to local policies and their application to nursing practice, with guidelines on practice, should be included to ensure safety for the nurse and patient. Broad general policies will be given for use in most clinical situations, and they will be related to safe practice. These might include infection control, health and safety and drug administration.

Infection control

Most Health Authorities employ an infection control specialist nurse. This does not mean however that nurses can abdicate their responsibility for control of infection, particularly in the wards. Although much infection control can be attributed to plain common sense and good nursing practice, this must be underwritten by sound rationale and research evidence rather than myth and tradition.

A basic understanding of the chain of infection and where and how this chain may be broken or interrupted by the nurse, forms the basis on which the principles of infection control are built. This understanding might prevent the following reported incidents from happening:

(1) Nurses ringing up the infection control nurse in panic saying that a patient they have admitted or are admitting has an infectious disease, and what should they do?
(2) Nurses stating they have a patient suffering from pulmonary tuberculosis so they are reverse barrier nursing her.
(3) Advising a patient who was told by his doctor he was suffering from shingles and was contagious, not infectious, who then refused to touch anything or go out in case other people caught the disease.

One needs to know that an infectious disease is caused by a micro-organism which has entered the body, overcome resistance and grown and multiplied. The source of the infection can be another infectious person or animal or an inanimate object that has been in contact with the micro-organism. Transmission of the micro-organism will therefore be from person to person or by touching a contaminated object or contact with the animal.

To prevent the spread of infection good nursing practices must be adhered to. Thorough hand washing and careful drying is an essential practice at all times. Attention must be paid to the cleansing of the environment and to disinfecting equipment in contact with the patient. Safe disposal of waste materials is essential. Barrier nursing may be required, either to protect the patient from infection or to protect others from being infected by a compromised patient.

Health and safety at work

Most nurses are aware of the Health and Safety at Work Act 1974. The importance of this Act in relation to nursing practice is two-fold.

Part of the responsibility under the Act lies with the employer and part with the employee. The main principle of the Act is that people are not harmed during the course of their work and that employees do not harm others by working. The most obvious examples would be that the employer reduces or removes the risk of employees coming into contact with hazardous substances such as radiation, chemicals, drugs, or infections such as hepatitis or tuberculosis. Employees reduce or remove the risk of endangering others by ensuring the work environment is safe by removing or covering trailing leads, not blocking exits or corridors with equipment and not bringing infections into the workplace.

There is also an obligation on employers and employees to make sure suitable training and supervised practice is instituted when and where appropriate, e.g. training people to lift and handle objects safely.

All employees need to know what to do in case of fire. Most institutions include fire drill in inductions of all new staff, with a regular annual up-date. It is the responsibility of staff to ensure they receive the necessary training.

Prevention of back injury

There is no doubt that all nurses are at risk of injuring their backs in the course of their work. Prevention of back injury must have a high priority in any preparation for the returning nurse.

Once again the responsibility is two-fold. The employer must provide a safe work environment where there is space and equipment to reduce or eliminate manual lifting. Also training is required to ensure employees know how to use the equipment. Employees need to be aware that they only have one back, which is their responsibility. They should understand the risks involved and not expose themselves to unnecessary hazards. They need to ensure that they are familiar with and confident in the accepted practices in their chosen area of work, and if there is any doubt they should ask for help and refuse to be involved until they feel competent. They also need to make sure they are fit to do the job required and that they maintain that fitness.

Drug administration

For most returning nurses a big source of anxiety about going into the clinical areas is administration of drugs, as mentioned in Chapter 3. This fear stems from a belief that 'all' drugs have changed and the returner will have to start from scratch to learn them all again. There is also an insecurity about the mathematical ability to work out drug doses. There is far less concern about drug administration and security. One returning nurse did observe that drugs were now stored in a locked trolley which was wheeled around the ward; 'what luxury' was her comment.

Most Health Authorities have a written Code of Conduct for safe drug administration. This is based on the premise that nurses have a professional duty to fulfil the doctor's prescription, ensuring the patient is not harmed in the process. In order to do this it is recognized that nurses need knowledge of local drug policies, and of the drugs themselves including the therapeutic effects, side effects and drug incompatibilities. Nurses also need to know normal dosages and administration routes, and should be able to calculate drug doses, interpret prescription sheets and maintain accurate records.

The five 'rights' of drug administration are: the *right* medication, in the *right* dosage, to the *right* patient, by the *right* route at the *right* time.

Nurses who hold the drug keys also have responsibility for the correct storage and security of the drugs in their area of responsibility. They should be aware that some preparations deteriorate if stored at other than optimum temperature, and that most drugs have a limited shelf life.

As mentioned in earlier chapters the practice of routine drug rounds at set times is slowly being eliminated. With the changes in ward organization and nurses taking on responsibility for the total care of a group of patients, this care will include administering drugs or enabling the patients in certain circumstances to self administer their drugs. The responsibility for holding the keys and the security then becomes more diffuse, requiring more vigilance and attention to detail.

Learning needs

Because returning nurses are individual in both their previous experiences and where they are going to work, one cannot generalize in what their learning needs will be during their clinical practice. Only the returners themselves can really state what they need to practise to regain their confidence and competence. They will however need some help and guidance initially in identifying what is possible and practicable in a given situation. One returning nurse to a surgical ward identified the following areas in which she needed practice:

- Admission of a patient and writing and using care plans.
- Pre- and post-operative care of a patient.
- Removal of clips, drains and sutures.
- Aseptic technique.
- Giving of medication, including intravenous fluids, pain relief and intramuscular injections.
- Fluid and food intake.
- Patient mobilization.
- Care of colostomy/ileostomy.

Clinical practice

There is no doubt that all students on the Return to Nursing course value very highly the opportunity to work on the wards as part of the course. The following statements by students verify this:

- 'Clinical practice was definitely a high spot and it was only then that I felt, yes, this is definitely me. I was delighted to have experienced more than one clinical area.'
- 'The opportunity for practical experience has been excellent and of tremendous value in renewing one's skills, catching up on modern methods of treatment and boosting one's confidence.'
- 'One might not have the courage to pursue clinical work if this hurdle was not overcome at this stage.'
- 'Going on to any ward breaks the ice and after ten weeks I feel so much more confident.'
- 'Gradually, with ward experience, I have gained more knowledge and confidence in the new nursing role.'
- 'I found the practical work aspect very helpful.'
- 'At first I thought the "new" approach was not for me, but after completing the clinical practice I found it was.'

Mentor system

The most important, common factor which made the clinical experience both enjoyable and a satisfactory learning opportunity was the mentor system. This meant that each student had an identified qualified nurse who was responsible for them throughout the course and was friend, counsellor, advisor and assessor. In addition the student was supernumerary, so there was time and opportunity not only to learn but also to make a contribution to the workforce as skills were regained.

The value of this system of mentorship and being supernumerary was frequently commented on by students:

- 'The practical work on the ward was very beneficial in being able to observe without too much responsibility.'
- 'I think the opportunity to observe then regain nursing skills under supervision, with the willingness and co-operation of all the ward staff, has been a very positive experience for me. My mentor also seemed to have a clear idea of how to approach my "retraining" and was very encouraging, offering me increased responsibilities or a variety of opportunities with each duty.'
- 'Both my mentors were highly professional nurses who always considered the quality of care for their patients and fostered a professional attitude with other members of the ward team.'

- 'It was useful having a mentor; I felt less vulnerable.'
- 'The ward situation was useful and the safe feeling of "the mentor" was comforting.'
- 'It was good to:
  - Be attached to a mentor.
  - Be supernumerary.
  - Be able to organize hours to suit one's lifestyle.
  - Have a practical day in the introductory block.

Problems of clinical practice

It would be misleading to suggest that all problems in returning to nursing were resolved by making the returner supernumerary and attaching her to a mentor in the chosen area. Problems still arose with procedure, equipment and the sheer logistics of organizing and co-ordinating time at work with family and personal commitments and time when the mentor was available, as the following comments demonstrate.

- 'I have found difficulty at work identifying all the various procedure packs since one has no idea whether they are large, small, fat or thin, or what any named pack actually contains. I end up starting at the top of the store and pulling out one of everything until I find something vaguely connected with what I want.'
- 'I always spent time soul searching about which technique to use doing dressings etc. But as long as you have a sound basic knowledge on aseptic technique, then it is up to you, the nurse, because you are fully accountable for your actions. I feel more relaxed and can enjoy my nursing more.'
- 'My weak areas are usage of drugs and care plans – from the point of view of making sure all relevant care is included for the patient, physical, mental and spiritual.'
- 'The nursing process and care plans were the biggest problems on returning to work.'
- 'The practical work was helpful but it so difficult to arrange suitable times as the allocated mentors were on night duty or on holiday when I could work.'
- 'It was difficult to arrange practical work although my staff nurse came in twice on her off-duty time.'

Criticism of both the preparation and placement included:

- 'More practical teaching involving nursing procedures would have helped.'

- 'More time should be given to actual treatments and techniques now in use on wards.'
- 'Clinical practice was very useful although I am sure more time on a busier surgical or medical ward would have benefited me.'
- 'One or two ward teaching sessions, visiting wards in groups, would have benefited us all greatly.'

Warm reception

Almost without exception, the reception the returners received in the clinical areas when they commenced the course, was warm and friendly. For most nurses this was unexpected but very much appreciated, as indicated by their comments:

- 'The ward was welcoming and clean, with a lovely atmosphere.'
- 'The staff were wonderful; there was a friendly atmosphere.'
- 'The staff were not busy, the ward was clean and there was a friendly bustle.'
- 'I was welcomed and put at ease.'
- 'There was a good atmosphere and liaison was good with a detailed report given, followed by a comprehensive orientation.'

Orientation

Besides the warm welcome, most returners were given an orientation or induction to the clinical area to which they were allocated. The orientation varied in its length and content from a brief showing around then being left 'to one's own devices', to a detailed report followed by a tour of the hospital, including the mortuary in one instance. Many commented on the fact that they were introduced to other members of NHS staff, which they felt was a great improvement from their day. The dietician and physiotherapist spent many hours on the ward, making the returner feel that they were part of a team caring for the patients. This team spirit was also mentioned by another returner:

'I was present at many discussions on how to improve the quality of care to the patient and how to improve communications between the members of the multidisciplinary team.'

However, all did not always run smoothly; even with the most careful preparation, when dealing with people the unexpected will happen, as these comments show:

- 'Following my initiation back into the practical field by a patient collapsing at my feet, I realized life had not changed to that great an extent and I could cope.'
- 'I had joined the handover report at the nurses station. I was asked if I would take the pulse and blood pressure of a patient opposite the station. It was several minutes later when I rather shamefacedly reported that I could not find a pulse. The lady had quietly died; I thought I had lost my skills!'

Staff attitudes

Most returners were overcome by the attitude of all the staff towards them. In addition to the friendliness already mentioned, they noted that:

> 'Everyone was so helpful and encouraging. I was also amazed at the informality both with nurses and other members of the health care team.'

One nurse reported that she was introduced to the consultant who warmly shook her hand and said how delighted he was that she had returned to nursing. The returners also commented how they enjoyed being with other nurses and several remarked on the pleasure of leaving home to return to work. They felt the adrenalin beginning to flow again.

One or two did however feel superfluous initially, and thought that with so many qualified nurses around it felt too comfortable and familiar. Indeed most commented on the fact that basic nursing care had not changed. Even the shabby old ward somehow perpetuated the impression that time had stood still while they were away, and in many areas things were not so up-to-date as they had been expecting.

Classroom practice

One of the biggest problems in organizing a Return to Nursing course is knowing to what degree and in what detail practical nursing skills should be included in the classroom teaching. This can be a problem even for those teaching basic nursing students. Because of the rapid changes in equipment and the range of methods of working employed in the clinical areas, no teachers can feel truly confident that what they are teaching in the classroom is necessarily what the nurse will find in the clinical area. This is further complicated with returning nurses who may well have been taught many different ways of performing an activity and will be returning to a wide variety of clinical situations.

One can of course sympathize with the nurse who, when doing something simple and basic like taking a temperature, was confronted with a thermometer which only registered just over 40°. The nurse was not aware that temperatures are now measured on the Celcius scale, the 'norm' being 37°. She was only familiar with the Fahrenheit scale where the 'norm' was 98.4°.

Similarly, there was the nurse who spent much valuable time looking for a back-rest for the bed when in fact all she had to do was wind the head of the bed up, and the nurse whose hands were shaking so much when she was trying to fill the syringe prior to giving an intramuscular injection, that her mentor had to leave the treatment room while she regained her composure.

Although this dilemma over what to teach them was explained to the returners both before and at the start of the course, it did little to alter their expectations. Probably because of previous training methods and apprehensions about their competence to perform clinical skills, it was clear most of them would have appreciated practical demonstrations in the classroom and the opportunity to try out some procedures, as shown by their comments in the evaluations at the end of the course:

- 'To have a classroom situation for ward procedures and how they are carried out would have been helpful. To have a real lifting session for patients would be a good idea, where students could use the aids which are used on the wards.'
- 'I would like to have been shown or told about the new types of everyday equipment in use, i.e. disposable thermometers and digital read-out blood pressure machines.'
- 'I would have appreciated more in-class practical tuition as part of the introductory block, e.g. blood pressure monitoring, temperature, pulse, respiration record keeping.'
- 'I would have liked to 'have a go' at lifting each other, with care, and using hoists in the classroom.'

There is no doubt that returning nurses exhibit a whole variety of fears and anxieties at the prospect of returning to the clinical areas to work. They tend to create a mystique for themselves from long past experiences and from more recent disjointed accounts from others. With careful, thoughtful preparation, based on experience and knowledge from those who have made the transition from home to work, together with a system of support, encouragement and protection, it is possible to make the return to nursing not only a pleasure but a positive experience which will sustain the returner through the difficulties ahead.

Further reading

Books

Chilman, A.M. & Thomas, M. (1987) *Understanding Nursing Care*, 3rd edn. Churchill Livingstone, Edinburgh.

Dugas, B.W. (1977) *Introduction to Patient Care*. W.B. Saunders, Philadelphia.

Watson, J.E. (1979) *Medical-Surgical Nursing and Related Physiology*. W.B. Saunders, Philadephia.

Oxfordshire Health Authority policies on:
- Prevention of Back Injury – Policy Note 20.
- Infection Control.
- Drug Code of Practice.
- Health & Safety.

Part 4
Forward to the Future

Chapter 8
Do I Still Want to Return?

If all the qualified nurses resident in this country were to return to full time professional practice, there would be no shortage, no need that could not be filled. Why then are the estimated 80 000 to 90 000 qualified nurses not returning to practise their profession?

In Chapter 3 we examined what motivated nurses to leave a comfortable secure world, over which they have some measure of control, to enter an insecure, frightening environment which had become alien to them. Many returners opt if possible for some kind of retraining, updating or refreshing programme before they take the final step into permanent paid employment. It is not uncommon however in the field of adult education for course members to end up rejecting the very work for which they were training. There is nothing like the real world for making people face up to reality. The nurse has to practise in the real world and needs to learn to practise with confidence and understanding, as confirmed by comments from two returners:

- 'The course has enabled me to judge realistically my situation. A gradual, lower-keyed "re-insertion" seems appropriate – probably a smaller local hospital situation to gain more experience.'
- 'The course has crystallized my thoughts and feelings on where I would be best suited to nurse.'

Staff shortages

One of the most frequently mentioned anxieties of the returners centred around staffing – not only lack of quantity but also lack of quality.

Staff shortages were recognized as being important because of the widespread stress and frustration they caused at all levels. Understaffing affected the morale of the remaining staff trying to give a good service, and also affected the smooth running of the ward or service. Many returners also felt that shortages of staff created a 'bad' ward atmosphere, with staff becoming impatient and unappreciative of any help. It also led to absenteeism and high staff turnover. Nurses are

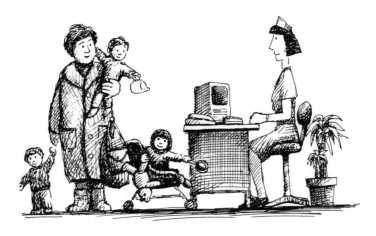

When can you start?

inclined to vote with their feet when the demands of the job become too great to bear.

Staffing problems also led to difficulties for the returner. First, it was sometimes impossible to place them in a clinical area of their choosing because there was not a sufficiently experienced nurse to act as a mentor; secondly, some returners suffered the frustration of their mentor leaving during their placement, which meant they had to be passed on to someone else who might not have the same interest or commitment to the student.

Some returners also felt that they had too much responsibility passed on to them too soon and very often had to learn from students or unqualified staff or manage themselves as best they could. This situation clearly did not encourage those who experienced it to take up employment at the end of the course.

As mentioned in Chapter 5 another effect of shortage of staff was the closure of beds and sometimes wards. This state of affairs was distressing to many returners, especially those who became directly involved when the ward to which they had been allocated was suddenly closed with little or no warning.

Skill mix

Skill mix in nursing has become a much discussed issue. Some argue for an all qualified nursing workforce giving direct patient care, while others feel this is not possible or even desirable in some circumstances. With changes in the organization of nursing care leading to the wider use of primary nursing and team nursing instead of task allocation, returners find it difficult to know where they fit into the scheme of things. They feel that with the disappearance of the student nurse, replaced by an all-trained staff, there is a lack of stimulation on the ward. They find too that there is no clear direction on how enrolled nurses and nursing auxiliaries should be used. One returner stated that:

'Nursing establishment levels fell below safe standards of practice when two nursing auxiliaries were in charge of a ward for the evening shift.'

Organization of work

On the other hand many nurses find it difficult to understand the role of the ward sister in a primary nursing or team nursing system, when the day to day management of the patients is in the hands of several qualified staff. One nurse was appalled that the ward sister did not know the names of all the patients. Others felt that without any central organization, care became muddled with no direction. Many related this situation to apparently poor nursing practices and poor standards of care.

Differences between theory and practice

They identified discrepancies between theory and practice which became even more acute when staffing levels were reduced. Then, because the 'proper' way usually took more time, the realistic way was adopted because it was quicker. This became apparent in lifting patients when a quick hitch under the arm, rather than using a mechanical hoist or the correct technique, achieved the end result far more quickly, despite the known risks to patient and nurse. Meals would often be left untouched by the patients, either because the food was unsuitable or because patients could not manage by themselves.

Although returners applauded the general philosophy that patients should be encouraged to do more for themselves, this should not be interpreted by the nurses that they can opt out of basic care.

There also appeared to be an inconsistency of recording in care plans which often led to an discontinuity of care. For instance if a catheter was removed or inserted, or if an intravenous infusion was discontinued, this information was not always indicated in the care plan, often leaving the nurse to find out by accident, as with one returner:

'One evening, according to the care plan, I was required to carry out pre-operative preparation for one patient who was due for major surgery the following day. When I approached the patient and explained what was about to happen he looked puzzled. I asked him why, only to hear that this had all happened that afternoon, including the enema. Needless to say I withdrew in great confusion. I cannot imagine the patient felt very confident in our ability to care for him.'

Discontentment with the system

Although a majority of returners felt reasonably comfortable with the changes in the system of delivering nursing care, there was a small minority who expressed discontent with the system. They felt uneasy with the practice of keeping care plans at the bottom of the bed, where patients and visitors could read them. They also did not like the increase in paperwork and form filling.

Returners had a general feeling of helplessness due to the changes in the system and not knowing the ward, patients or the routine. Some too felt frustration at being unable to change a routine or system with which they disagreed. What they did however recognize was that nursing remained a demanding, stressful, responsible job and one which they could not walk away from. This led to conflict with home interests as two nurses recounted:

- 'My husband insisted on meeting me after the evening shift. I finally got off duty at 10 PM, to be greeted by the comment, "If that is nursing, forget it!"'
- I was due to finish my shift in the next half hour, when the hospital was put on red alert because of a major incident. I had to wait a further two hours before I was cleared to go. My family had to manage without me.'

Pay and conditions of service

Pay and conditions of service are not very often mentioned by returners. This might be explained by the fact that many returners come from the age when nursing was seen as a vocation, where people entered and re-entered because they wanted to be of service to others. Also they are concerned that pay should not improve to the point where the wrong type of person might come into nursing.

Grading structure

The introduction of the grading structure, together with pay increases negotiated by a pay review body, has firmly linked pay with promotion and the creation of a career structure in clinical nursing. This of course needs explaining to returners who read job advertisements for D Grade or F Grade staff nurses and wonder what this means.

Under the old system, if nurses wanted to improve their remuneration they were often forced to make a decision between staying at the bedside on a lower salary or moving into administration or education away from direct patient contact. The grading structure allows the nurse to remain at the bedside but move to a higher grading, and therefore a higher salary, by offering qualifications and skills to improve patient care and the service given. This might be, for example, by teaching the patient and staff knowledge and skills in a particular area of care; by taking on responsibility for a particular area of administration, such as the duty roster; by carrying out nursing research to improve or enhance care; or by being a mentor for students training in that area.

Although there are obvious advantages to such a scheme there are also disadvantages, and the system has not been universally welcomed or liked. Some problems have been caused by a misunderstanding of the system by its administrators and recipients. In some less scrupulous organizations a higher grade has been used as a bribe to attract staff from elsewhere.

In the old hierarchical system if nurses stayed long enough in a post, and were therefore experienced, they assumed that when a post for promotion became vacant they would automatically be considered and would be likely to secure the post. Now they have to demonstrate that they have not only experience but also suitable qualifications, which usually means undertaking some kind of professional development. Much of the discontent over the new grading structure arose from the fact that many staff in fairly senior positions did not merit them either by the work they did, the responsibilities they held or the further training or development they had undertaken over the preceding years.

Most enrolled nurses are placed on a C grade and most RGNs are placed on a D grade. Each grade has incremental points. To move up the grades nurses usually have to negotiate with their managers. Occasionally some enrolled nurses are on D grade and a rare few will be on E grade when they can demonstrate a particularly high level of knowledge and expertise in a special area of nursing. Unfortunately, however, if they leave that area of nursing they might well go back to C grade.

Most part-time staff will be on the basic grade because, it is argued, they do not work enough hours to merit a higher grade. In some areas however if part-time nurses can show that the job demands nurses with their qualifications and expertise, they might be awarded a higher grade.

Incentives/disincentives

Although the salary is important to any returning nurse, there are other factors which may influence the decision to take a job. It is recognized that there are very few incentives in nursing such as a car, sports facilities, free meals, or help with housing or subsidized holidays. It is however the financial costs which are more important to the returning nurse in deciding whether it is worthwhile returning at all. The two main costs will be travel to work and childcare expenses.

Travel

Not all nurses can drive or will have access to a car. The car might have to be shared with a partner, which will take some careful organization about who has the car and the starting and finishing times for work. Costs of petrol and parking, and the availability of parking, will have to be considered. If a car is not available, public transport costs and times will have to be calculated when checking outlay for work. This becomes even more critical when the returner works only part-time or on a casual basis. Travel costs can consume a large part of one's salary.

Childcare

The need for childcare provision is neither recognized nor accepted by many Health Service employers. Even when crêche and holiday playschemes exist the costs have to be met by the user. When there are one or two children in the family, and possibly only one wage earner, the cost can be prohibitive to the point where the financial rewards for working do not exist. One nurse explained why she was giving up work she enjoyed:

> 'I travel 30 miles each way to work. I have four children under nine for whom I employ a nanny. By the time I have deducted all my expenses I end up paying the NHS for the privilege of working for them. I can no longer afford this.'

Flexible hours

For many returners the only way they can get the flexible working hours to suit their domestic circumstances is to do bank or agency nursing. This will limit the scale at which they are paid and job promotion opportunities. Also, they will not receive any sick pay or paid holidays nor will they qualify for redundancy money or employment pension. Income tax and National Insurance contributions will be automatically deducted however if their earnings meet the required level. In addition there is no job security and no guarantee that work will be available where and when required. The problems this can cause were graphically illustrated by one returner I met some time after she had completed the course:

'As a one parent family with three children and no other means of support and help I thought a return to nursing was the answer. With no means of transport other than an erratic bus service my only option was to work in the nearby local community hospital. As I could only offer school hours in which to work it was suggested I did bank work. All was well for several months, then the hospital ran out of money in its nursing budget. There was no work available, I could not travel, I did not qualify for the dole, and I was thrown back on to social security. It was very hard after having a reasonable income for some time.'

Job security and status

Job security and a measure of self esteem help returning nurses regain confidence and build competence in their work. However, those who manage the workforce do not appear always actively to assist nurses who wish to return to nursing.

The aspirations of returners in relation to status are seldom met. Although a few returners can manage full time work with its irregular and often unsocial hours, a majority are obliged to work part-time and therefore have to accept possible demotion and downward mobility.

For example, one returner had previously held a senior, responsible position as a sister in charge of an intensive care department but could only expect to obtain the post of a staff nurse part-time on a general ward. Another returner was formerly a clinical teacher in a renal unit. As clinical teachers were no longer employed she was obliged to work on a medical ward as a staff nurse until she was in a position to pick up the threads of teaching again.

Both these returners felt undervalued and underused with having to take orders from very junior staff who often knew much less than they did.

Age range

It is felt by many that nursing still worships at the altar of youth, especially in the large general hospitals. Indeed, one manager of the nursing workforce of such a hospital has stated that of his 750 nursing staff about three quarters were single women under 25 years of age. He could count on one hand part-time mature staff and on two hands the number of male nurses that were working there.

Of course the whole system was geared to the single young person working full time with an unbroken career. Work was organized with internal rotation to night duty and most wards used primary or team nursing as a method of delivering care. As a prestigious hospital there was never a problem of recruitment even though there was a constant movement of nurses.

One can only wonder how long this situation can be perpetuated and how the hospital will cope when its current source of staffing begins to dry up. Because there is little or no demand there are no allowances made for married women and parents.

Bank and agency nursing

As demands for childcare facilities and flexible and part-time work are not met, the only option for returners who want to work in the acute admitting hospital will be bank or agency nursing. This is of course less than ideal for people who lack confidence. The feeling of not belonging anywhere, not knowing where they are working and being treated as an outsider and with suspicion makes them feel very insecure. Many give up the unequal struggle and turn to other occupations such as offices, shops, pubs and factories.

As can be seen, trying to plan a return to the nursing workforce can be fraught with difficulties, but for the determined and strong-minded it is possible:

'If you think you are beaten, you are.
If you think you dare not, you don't.
If you'd like to win, but think you can't
it's most certain you won't.
For out of this world we find
success begins with a fellow's will –
It's all in the state of mind.'

Anon

What work do I want?

For the fortunate few who appear in the right place at the right time there is no problem, as they are snapped up by a desperate management; like the nurse who just popped round to the local nursing home to make enquiries and was asked to start that evening; or the returner with theatre experience who, while doing her clinical placement on a surgical ward, was quizzed by the theatre staff when she took a patient to theatre. When they found out who she was and what experience she had, she was asked to see the theatre superintendent who offered her a job there and then at hours to suit her convenience.

For most returners however there is a need to think about what they want to achieve when choosing a job, and to develop an appropriate strategy. Some people return to work first, then decide later what they want to do. It makes far more sense however to give some thought to more than just fulfilling immediate needs, to avoid possible disappoint-

	Responsibilities	What I did	What I enjoyed most	What I enjoyed least
Education & training				
Employment				
Special skills/leisure				

Fig. 8.1 Personal assessment of achievements and abilities.

ment at a later date. As a fair number of hours may be spent at work it is reasonable to enjoy what is done there.

Self assessment – What can I do?

A good starting point for developing any job searching strategy is to start with yourself: to assess as objectively as possible your achievements and abilities and to recognize weaknesses and aversions. One way of accomplishing this is to list information about yourself. Record first details of education and training, then employment experience and finally special skills and leisure interests. You might make comments by your entries regarding any responsibilities you assumed, what you actually did and what you enjoyed most or least. See Fig. 8.1 for an example.

Goals

Having completed an assessment it is worth spending some time considering what job you are looking for. Note down the work you are experienced in, even if it was many years ago. What level of responsibility are you aiming for? Try not to be too modest. Are you mainly interested in clinical nursing or are you more attracted to management or teaching? Have you considered the grade you will be placed on and do you know what incremental point you will be awarded? See Fig. 8.2 for salary scales from April 1992. Have

Standard payroll system code	Pay grade Title/scale	Min. £	1 £	2 £	3 £	4 £	5 £	6 £	Pay spine Points
					Incremental points				
NP01	Scale A (age point) Under age 18	6400							
NP06	Scale A	Point 3 7000	7250	7500	7760	8030	8300	8570	3–9
NP16	Scale B	Point 8 8300	8570	8840	9140	9450			8–12
NP21	Scale C	Point 12 9450	9770	10100	10460	10820	11180		12–17
NP26* NP31*	Scale D	Point 16 10820	11180	11580	11990	12400			16–20
NP36	Scale E	Point 20 12400	12810	13250	13750	14350			20–24
NP41	Scale F	Point 23 13750	14350	14960	15580	16200	16830		23–28
NP46	Scale G	Point 27 16200	16830	17460	18100	18750			27–31
NP51	Scale H	Point 30 18100	18750	19400	20050	20700			30–34
NP56	Scale I	Point 33 20050	20700	21360	22030	22700			33–37

* Use of pay codes: Pay code NP26 should be assigned to second level (enrolled) nurses, and Pay code NP31 to first level (registered) nurses including nurses holding the certificate of the British Thoracic Association.

This information is required for manpower planning purposes.

Fig. 8.2 Nursing and midwifery staffs' pay scales effective from 1 April 1992 – clinical grading structure. The pay scales form part of the Nursing and Midwifery Staff's Negotiating Council Conditions of Service and Rates of Pay (ISBN 1 85197 156 4).

you discussed with your family how your work will affect them and what sacrifices they might have to make? How ambitious are you? What can you realistically aim for now and what are you hoping to achieve in the future?

Personal details

The final stage in assessment is to consider the personal factors which will influence your choice of work:

(1) *Marital status* Will the fact that you are single, married, divorced, separated or widowed place restrictions on job opportunities; e.g. if you are married and your husband travels a lot you cannot rely on him to care for the children on a regular basis. Or as stated earlier if you share a car and he needs it to go to work early in the morning you might not be able to do night work.

(2) *Dependants* These could be children, parents, relatives or friends. What are their demands on your time, attention and money? Will these influence where and when and if you work at all?

(3) *Finance* We all have fixed and variable financial commitments. Have you considered the minimum income on which you can exist? What do you feel is desirable?

(4) *Health* What is your energy capacity? Are you prone to illnesses? Do you have allergies or handicaps? How much stress and strain can you take in your work? Are you physically capable of a full day's work plus? Nursing today is very demanding both physically and mentally. You need to be fit and active.

(5) *Age* Many returners are anxious about their age, fearing it may prevent them from being selected for a job. There is no upper age limit imposed by the UKCC for registration to practise as a nurse. The NHS will allow nurses to work up to the age of 65, yet two thirds of the nursing workforce is under the age of 40. There are few official limitations regarding age, although health may have a part to play in any decision. I have seen many returners in their fifties make a successful return and I knew of one woman making enquiries who was 68 years old.

Having now spent some time considering what you have to offer and what you need in the way of work, you are ready to move to the next stage in your strategy: looking at the job market. There are many sources of information about work available for returning nurses.

What work is available?

Your local job centre receives details of vacancies daily, including those at local hospitals and nursing homes. They can also help you find the right kind of work to suit you and can advise about training opportunities and other schemes which may be able to help you. There are also private recruitment agencies specifically for nurses. They will know of both local and national needs and some have an international brief for recruitment. These usually charge a fee to either the employer or employee or both. Look in the Yellow Pages for their addresses and telephone numbers.

Job advertisements

Advertisements for nursing posts are another obvious source of information about nursing vacancies. National newspapers will carry some advertisements, usually if there is a recruitment drive on or if private hospitals and homes are recruiting nationally. A more likely source for local hospitals will be local newspapers. You may also need to scan the professional journals, many of which carry several pages of job advertisements. Your local library could well have copies of both the papers and journals. Health centres, clinics and dental surgeries may also display job advertisements.

Read the advertisements critically as they may vary from two or three lines mentioning a vacancy for a staff nurse to a full page advertisement which includes details of the location of the hospital and the nature of the vacancy. This can indicate that the hospital placing the first advertisement was poor, or that the employer placing the second advertisement was desperate to attract staff.

If an advertisement appears attractive but does not match your qualifications or experience it is always worthwhile making enquiries. Most advertisements state what the employer would ideally prefer, but depending on how desperate they are they may be willing to negotiate on any aspects of the job the candidate lacks but would be willing to acquire.

Local hospitals

Not all vacancies are advertised outside the hospital, either because of the cost or because of repeated failure to fill a vacancy. It is always worthwhile therefore visiting or telephoning your local hospital or nursing home to make enquiries. In fact, this is usually the most common way nurses find out what is happening locally.

It is the kind of reception nurses receive at this stage which can be crucial in successfully attracting them back into the workplace. A rude or ill-informed secretary or telephonist can do more damage to a hesitant, unsure nurse making enquiries than any bad experiences that the nurse has had nursing in the past. It is worth persisting and asking to see and talk to the personnel nurse or nurse manager, who will have an overall view of current job vacancies and the future needs of the hospital. They might also advise on courses available to returners and 'in touch' programmes so that contact is not lost. They will also know the hospital's attitude to part-time, flexible and job sharing possibilities for the mature nurse, and they might explain the various job titles and grades and their relation to practice.

Word of mouth

Next to ringing or visiting the local hospital word of mouth is the most common way for nurses to find out about local hospital provision and job opportunities. Wherever groups of women meet – in leisure pursuits, doing the shopping or meeting the children from school – experiences are recounted which encourage the listener to make further enquiries. One nurse I met recently, who had made a successful return to nursing two years ago, recalled how it all started:

'One morning I was feeling particularly low and depressed; it seemed life had nothing to offer me. I was coming up to 40 years of age, the children were happy in school, my husband was absorbed in his work, but all I had was housework and shopping. I felt old and rejected. I bumped into a friend who was in similar circumstances to me but she was looking bright and energetic. She told me she had returned to district nursing and was loving every minute of it, and she wondered why I didn't return. I went home, rang the hospital and have not looked back since. It was the beginning of a whole new life. I have slowly increased my hours as family commitments allowed and I am now going on to do the diploma in nursing.'

Whichever way you have found out about a job vacancy the next stage in your strategy is to apply for a job and if selected attend an interview.

Job application

To apply for a job you may telephone, write a letter or fill out an application form, or any combination of all three. This stage can be crucial in the whole procedure. How you present yourself on the telephone, how you write your letter and even what paper you use, and how you fill in the application form will influence the prospective employer on your suitability for the job.

Telephone call

Preparation is important in all three instances. When you make a telephone call, make sure you have time and money to do so. Reduce interruptions and background noises to the minimum so that you can hear and be heard. Screaming, fighting children or loud music in the background will not impress any employer. Tell them what you have to offer, how you think you will be an asset to them and get them to make a decision. Agree and confirm what happens next: a meeting, informal visit, interview, put on the waiting list or call again. Make a note of what is said and follow up with a letter confirming this.

Letter writing

When writing a letter, whether it is to ask if there are any vacancies, to apply for a job, or ask for an application form, keep it short and to the point. Type it if your handwriting is not legible, and use plain undecorated paper, not that torn from a spiral bound notepad or decorated with flowers or animals or cartoons. I have seen many of these binned without a second glance.

Application forms

Application forms frighten many people and are as a consequence poorly completed. General guidelines are:

- Read the instructions thoroughly.
- Do a rough copy first.
- Make sure you answer the questions asked.
- Write neatly and tidily, using a black pen (some employers now accept typed applications).
- Don't cramp your writing; use another sheet of paper if necessary.
- Make sure you post the form back before the closing date for applications.
- Keep a copy of what you have written.

The information you have already collected about yourself will be very useful in your application.

The interview

As with the application, preparation is all important for the interview. Find out as much about the hospital, nursing home or department as you can. How big is it? How many staff work there? What kind of patients are cared for? Find out as much about the work as possible. What are you likely to be doing? What will they want from you? What are the pay and conditions? What do you have to offer this particular job? What skills and experiences are most relevant? What are you likely to be asked? What work have you done in the past? Why are you looking for work now? Why have you applied for this particular job? Would you be willing to be trained? When can you start? What can I ask them? More about the job? More about the hospital or department?

Sort out how you will get to the interview and how long it will take to get there. Make sure you have all the documents you need. Sort out what you are going to wear: be neat and tidy.

At the interview:

- Be on time, or if anything a little early to give you time to relax.
- Be polite; do not sit until invited.
- Listen and answer the questions you are being asked, avoiding yes and no answers.
- Talk at your usual pace and tone; try not to mumble or stray from the question.
- Think about the question; if you do not understand what is asked, ask the interviewer to explain.
- Find out how a decision will be made and how and when you will be told.
- At the end of the interview say 'thank you' and leave. Don't hang about.

If you are successful, congratulations and good luck in your new job. If you are unsuccessful do not let it stop you looking for and applying for other jobs. Ask the interviewers why you did not get the job; tell them you would like to know for future reference. Patience and persistence may be required if a successful outcome is to be achieved.

'You've got to think high to rise.
You've got to be sure of yourself before
You can ever win a prize.
Sooner or later the man who wins
Is the one who thinks he can.'

Anon

Further reading

Books

Dean, D.J. (1987) *Manpower Solutions*. RCN/Scutari Press, London.

Lysaught, J.P. (1981) *Action in Affirmation – Toward an Unambiguous Profession of Nursing*. McGraw-Hill Co. (UK) Ltd.

Mackay, L. (1989) *Nursing A Problem*. Open University Press, Milton Keynes.

Woodcock, M. & Francis, D. (1989) (reprint) *The Unblocked Manager*. Gower, London.

Booklets

Job Hunting – information booklet. Manpower Services Commission. Available from Job Centres.

The Job-Hunting Handbook, Professional & Executive Recruitment edition. From Executive Post, Fitzwilliam Gate, Sheffield, S1 4JH.

Articles

Baker, J. Preparing a CV. *Nursing Times*, **85**(24) 56–8.

Place, B. (1989) How to augment your CV. *Nursing Standard*, **3**(18) 39.

Useful addresses

If you do want to consider working abroad the following are useful sources of information:

International Department
Royal College of Nursing
20 Cavendish Square
London W1M 0AB

Records and Registrations
UKCC for Nursing, Midwifery and
Health Visiting
23 Portland Square
London W1N 3AF

Chapter 9
Training and Professional Development

In today's world no one can complete an education. Continuing education is recognized as a critical component in the development of any professional. For it to be effective however there should be a systematic, planned approach to learning. This approach should be designed to promote the development of knowledge, skills and attitudes for the enhancement of nursing practice to improve the health care of the public. Basic nurse education can only be a foundation. It should prepare nurses for lifelong learning and should teach them to question their practice.

Nurse preparation

It was the view of the United Kingdom Central Council in the early 1980s that with the rapidly changing health and social needs of society there was a need to address the deficiencies in the present system of nurse preparation. It was felt that the system was inflexible and did not make the best use of human and financial resources. There had also been a groundswell of discontent from the profession with the apprenticeship type of training, and there were indications that such training could not be sustained indefinitely because:

(1) The decline in the number of 18-year-old school leavers from which student nurses are recruited will continue until the mid-1990s.
(2) Other occupations and professions will be competing more keenly for the smaller number of qualified school leavers.
(3) Overall one in five of all student nurses drop out or fail to register at the end of their course.
(4) One in ten qualified nurses leave the profession each year.

It was clear that major reforms were needed.

There had been much discussion over the years, both of the need for change and how this change could be effected. Reports were written and recommendations were made, notably the Briggs report

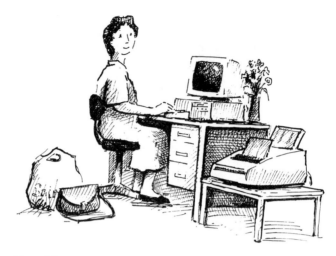

Return with confidence.

(1973) (see Further Reading). In the early 1980s however it was felt that although many of the arguments for change put forward by Briggs were still valid, the length of time that had elapsed, the developments which had intervened and the new operational structures pointed to a need for a fresh look at educational preparation for nursing.

Project 2000

In view of the mounting pressure for reform a committee was set up in 1985 by the UKCC to review the current situation, make recommendations and outline a strategy to achieve the changes required. After much deliberation a lengthy document was produced entitled *A New Preparation for Practice*, or Project 2000 as it became more commonly known. This document, together with videos, was widely disseminated throughout the profession for discussion and comment. Reactions were fed back to the committee for consideration. A series of supplementary documents was also produced to expand on and explain various aspects of the debate, such as student status and facing the future.

At a meeting in January 1987 the UKCC finally agreed its proposals for the reform of education and training, following the wide-ranging consultations with the professions and on the basis of consultancy work on manpower, finance and implementation. The proposals, summarized below, were not universally accepted, but all agreed that there was a need for improvement in educational preparation and therefore a willingness to accept the inevitable changes.

Supernumerary status

The first proposal stated that there would be a new single level of nurse who would embrace much of the work of the present two levels. This nurse would be a 'knowledgeable doer'. The competencies required of the nurse would be enshrined in statutory rules. They should include the ability to assess the need for, provide, monitor and evaluate care in both an institutional and non-institutional setting. Although in principle this was supported strongly by a majority, there were some serious doubts and reservations about the implications of such a proposal.

The doubts involved two other proposals: that the student should be supernumerary during education and training, and that enrolled nurse training should cease. As these groups represent a fair proportion of the workforce it was reasonable to ask who was going to replace them.

This was an issue that both the profession and the Government wanted addressed as a criterion for accepting the proposals. Recruitment and retention of staff, improving job satisfaction and maintaining standards of care all became part of the general debate.

The government stated that there should be strategic and operational plans for future manpower requirements, which were regularly reviewed. Further there should be systematic methods to agree the number and deployment of staff in all health care settings. Recruitment plans should pay particular attention to the needs of re-entrants, contacts should be maintained and conditions of service should be flexible so as to facilitate the return of those taking career breaks.

However, this message has yet to filter through to many managers who are still stating they do not want part-timers on their staff and will not even consider job-sharing. Thinking and planning ahead does not enter into their employment philosophy as evidenced by returners trying to get part-time or flexible working hours.

Cost

The cost of all these changes could not be ignored. It was proposed that the new students would no longer receive a salary as they were no longer part of the service, but should instead, like students in any higher education, receive a means-tested grant but controlled by the NHS. The funding thus released could be given back to the service side to employ alternative staff. Many will judge the government's commitment to Project 2000 by the provision of adequate funding.

Most agreed that the student should be supernumerary but their replacements should be qualified staff to ensure that teaching in the practical setting is properly achieved. Many returners in recent years have noted the high number of qualified nurses working in the clinical areas, compared with the one or two per shift when they last worked.

Support workers

One very controversial proposal that now has firm government backing and was in fact one of the conditions of accepting Project 2000, is the employment of a new range of unqualified helpers supervised by nurses. These helpers could be nursing assistants, nurses' aides, care assistants, support workers, nursing auxiliaries, health care support workers and others. The range of work they would do, and the training they would receive, is still causing strong feelings among the nursing profession.

As time passes it is becoming increasingly clear in some areas of the country and in some branches of nursing that there are not enough qualified nurses around to meet the demand for care. Even taking into consideration the growing opportunities for enrolled nurses to convert to first level nurse, there are still insufficient to meet the need. This, coupled with the government directive that all Health Authorities had to submit a plan for training the unqualified helper for national vocational qualifications, by spring 1991, forced nursing to seriously consider the issues; such as what work they should do, how they will be supervised and assessed, and by whom.

Programme framework

There were several proposals relating to the actual student nurse training programme. Although the details of the programme were missing the framework received guarded approval. First, it was agreed that the training and education of the new nurse should take three years, with the first 18 months consisting of a common foundation programme. This would be followed by an 18 month branch programme in mental health, mental handicap, midwifery, adult or children's nursing. Joint professional and academic validation should be sought and facilities should be no less than the best in higher education; at the same time the preparation should have a high practical content.

In addition, for general care, the European Directives (1977, 1989) for training programmes needed to be met to permit nurses to move from one EC country to another and achieve registration in any member state. The basic requirements are that programmes should last three years or 4600 hours and should consist of no less than one third theory and a half clinical instruction. The clinical instruction must be gained in general and specialist medicine, general and specialist surgery, maternity care, paediatrics, psychiatry, care of the elderly and care in the community.

Training environment

The education and training environment was also said to need improvement. Suggestions are that:

- The teacher:student ratio is 1:12;
- There is appropriate teacher education and orientation and an aim of a graduate teaching force;
- The practitioners in the clinical areas should receive formal preparation for their changing role;
- And facilities generally are in line with the best for higher education.

It was recognized that to achieve these improvements it might be necessary to concentrate and amalgamate current educational resources. As time has passed and Project 2000 is beginning to be implemented nationwide, the results are becoming more obvious to everyone involved. Individual schools of nursing are closing, and some are amalgamating with others in the same locality, making links with higher education and setting up as colleges of nursing.

Others are developing in different ways, for example Oxford has set up a Department of Health Care Studies based in the local Polytechnic and is running a four year Honours Degree course in Health Care Studies, with a professional qualification in nursing.

There is some regret and some misgiving in the profession about the loss of schools of nursing and about the emphasis on academic qualifications. The question asked is that, as nursing is essentially a practical occupation, will the new 'breed' of nurses want to give basic nursing care? The evidence is that from the degree training for nursing which has been taking place in the UK for the past 20 years, student wastage during training is lower, more of them stay at the bedside nursing than their RGN counterparts, and more are likely to go on in the profession and gain further nursing qualifications.

Post-registration education

The final group of proposals in Project 2000 centred around what happens after qualification. It is agreed and accepted by all that initial nursing education is the foundation stone of a professional career. There is however a need to learn and grow throughout one's professional life in order to give an effective service. Professional education therefore cannot be seen as a 'one-off' event at the beginning of one's career, but rather as a lifelong commitment to develop and learn. Included in the proposals must be a coherent, comprehensive framework of education beyond registration.

Approval for Project 2000

The full proposals of Project 2000 were finally submitted to the government in February 1987 and received approval in principle in May 1988. It is too early to determine whether outcomes have been achieved. Most parts of the country are in the early stages of implementation or preparation for implementation. That Project 2000 is going ahead in all four countries of the UK is a matter of some satisfaction.

But it has to be remembered that the reform of pre-registration education is only part of the story. As already mentioned, education and learning must be a continuous process throughout one's professional life. To this end the UKCC launched its post-registration education and practice project (PREPP) in early 1990.

PREPP

As with Project 2000, the outcomes of PREPP will have an effect on everyone with a nursing qualification, whether they are currently practising or not. The underlying aim of PREPP is not only to maintain standards of practice but also to improve them. In its Code of Professional Conduct (1984) the UKCC stated that:

> 'Each registered nurse, midwife and health visitor is accountable for his or her practice, and in the exercise of accountability shall . . . take every reasonable opportunity to maintain and improve professional knowledge and competence . . .'

Although this statement was not questioned or challenged by the profession generally, there was only minimal acceptance of the implications for most practitioners. For many nurses who qualified a decade or more ago and for many who are returning, the revelation that there is a need to up-date their practice is quite amazing. They were led to believe that their initial training and qualification were for their entire professional life and they knew all they needed to know to practise nursing.

Need for further education/training

As with nurse preparation, the need for change in education and training is indisputable both in professional and social terms. The changing health care needs, the shift of care from hospital to the community and the emphasis on prevention and health education, all represent major changes in the necessary skills and knowledge to practise safely. This is coupled with the fact that the general public is much more informed about health and the provisions made for any breakdown in health, and is therefore more demanding and critical.

It is no longer therefore appropriate for the decision for refreshment to be left to the discretion of the individual. Some element of compulsion was needed to encourage those who still practised in an uninformed way to comply with the Code of Professional Conduct.

This should not however lead to the following bitter comment from a student who had just completed such a course:

> 'I am glad I did the course, if only because to be employed you need it; past experiences do not count any more to employers, although we are led to believe they do.'

Terms of reference

A project group was set up to address these issues. Their brief was to identify the educational needs of nurses beyond registration; to make recommendations as to how professionals will maintain their competence and standards of practice; to identify levels of practice and training for those beyond registration; and finally to devise a framework to enable the standards, practice and education beyond registration to meet the needs of the public.

The challenge that this presents is that it has to be achieved within an ever-changing social environment. People are living longer, resulting in a growing elderly population. The birth rate is falling, therefore there will be fewer people around to care for the elderly. Technology has achieved an increased survival rate for the young and severely disabled who will need care all their lives.

There is an urgent need therefore to develop post basic programmes to enable qualified nurses to gain the additional skills and knowledge necessary to meet the new and expanding areas of care. As the RCN stated:

> 'Properly educated health professionals are not a sophisticated optional extra, but an essential prerequisite to efficient, effective health care.'

It follows therefore that it is essential that the qualified workforce acquires the skilled flexibility that will enable them to readily adapt to any changes. A thorough grounding in the latest clinical practice and a personal commitment to long term self-education to keep abreast of developments, are also necessary. What do nurses say about this responsibility?

> 'I have been made aware of the new nursing education programmes; how nursing is changing, very quickly. The course has given me the background information that I can expand on and has increased my desire to be part of nursing in the 1990s, contributing not witnessing.
>
> 'Many of the suggested ways to increase the soundness of our practice are good, but there are only 24 hours in a day! However, steadily keeping one's abilities up-to-date through reading, study and cross reference with colleagues is what to strive for.'

Objectives of training

The long term objectives of any continuing education programme should be for every qualified nurse to:

- Acquire relevant knowledge and perfect skills.
- Be able to implement and evaluate research findings.
- Explain and defend reasons for prescribing care.
- Understand the nurse's role in the wider health care team and be flexible.

These objectives will only be met if other issues are also addressed, such as:

- Career aspirations are understood.
- Regular training/educational opportunities are provided.
- Tangible benefits from training are forthcoming.
- The needs of nurses with family commitments are considered when designing such a programme.

Standards for practice

The project team took into consideration both the challenge and the objectives when advancing the discussion of maintaining standards for practice. It is understood and accepted that many practitioners will be happy to stay in the same sphere of work for their whole working lives. What is not acceptable is that there will therefore be no further need to train or study. As discussed in Chapter 5 on changes in nursing, the *status quo* is not an option. Experience alone will not necessarily maintain the level of competence at the registration standard point. The professional will need to expand and develop areas of professional expertise. This will of course depend on the clinical area, access to continuing education and the degree of commitment by the practitioner and the employer.

For those practitioners who seek to further their career, but not necessarily by upward moves or grooming for management positions, an advanced practitioner role is visualized. Many professionals today are more interested in moving towards a quality of life, broadening their experiences and continuing to build skill and knowledge, without moving up the ladder.

Theory/practice gap

One of the old 'chestnuts' in nursing education is the theory/practice gap: that practical and academic skills are seen as mutually exclusive.

This is coupled with the fear that as nurse preparation moves into higher education, practical nursing skills will suffer and the gap will widen even further, perhaps to irredeemable lengths. This of course is firmly rejected by Project 2000 planners who are required to include a statutory number of clinical hours in the preparation programme. (See the EC directives mentioned under 'Programme framework' earlier in this chapter.) Education beyond registration must be concerned with the quality of care that patients receive and must be relevant to the health care needs of society.

The new Project 2000 nurses will have a qualification at higher educational diploma level which will give them academic credibility. Existing practitioners who wish to aquire academic creditation for their qualifications can apply to Institutions of Higher Education for creditation. These will be awarded through the Credit Accumulation and Transfer Scheme (CATS) which is run by most Higher Educational Institutions. It is also felt strongly that credit accumulation should allow for experience to be recognized and included. This is now being offered by some Institutions through accreditation of prior experiential learning (APEL).

Review system

It is assumed by both the public and the profession that any nurse who holds a qualification will practise at the highest possible standard. The professional will only be able to offer a higher standard of practice however if they have been able to expand and develop their knowledge and expertise.

In order to achieve this it is suggested that a review system is established. This will ensure not only that there are opportunities for professional development but also that each professional has an individual responsibility to maintain and develop their own standards of practice. Such a system would need to be flexible to allow for changing health care needs and differing areas of practice. It should also be positive and possible for the professional to pursue.

Professional profile

One practical way of achieving these aims would be by the nurse providing and maintaining a professional profile. This would include evidence of learning activities and innovative practice or excellence in specific aspects of professional practice. Quite how evidence will be kept of the latter has yet to be decided. It is suggested that such a professional development profile will be a statutory requirement. It will be used both to identify learning which has taken place and to identify future learning needs. The profile should contain:

(1) A biographical sketch of experience to date.
(2) Statements of achievement on completion of studies or experiences.
(3) Developments in practice with an indication of the standard achieved and how this may be measured.

The question of whether the practitioner will, or should be given by right, a specific amount of study leave per annum in order to fulfil these requirements has yet to be decided. A system of self verification will be used for practitioners to confirm to the Council that its requirements have been met, on a three yearly basis when seeking to re-effect their registration. What has already been decided by the UKCC is that a specific return to a professional practice programme must be undertaken following a break in practice of five years or more. A review of development needs should also be undertaken.

Professional development

There is no doubt that with all the changes in nurse preparation and education, nursing practice is being substantially changed. Unfortunately, as has been suggested earlier, provision and uptake of post registration education is patchy throughout the country. This is of course a reflection of the attitude of both managers and staff to the need for and benefits of any professional development. This is in spite of the fact that as long ago as 1974 the American Nursing Association stated that:

> 'Planned learning experiences beyond registration should be designed to promote the development of knowledge skills and attitudes for the enhancement of nursing practice, thus improving health care to the public.'

This was echoed the following year in the statement of the International Congress of Nursing:

> 'Planned learning experiences beyond basic nurse education programmes should be designed to promote the development of knowledge, skills and attitudes for the enhancement of nursing practice, thus improving health care to the public.'

It follows therefore that professional development should mean continued growth, performance and reward for all staff who are motivated to develop their potential and performance. It has to be recognized that professional development is not necessarily that which occurs in classrooms and in formal training programmes. Most employees, when given the opportunity, can offer realistic suggestions for enriching their current work.

Working colleagues can have a strong impact on development. Formal teachers and outside agents may not always be in the best position to provide developmental experiences for professionals. One group of nurses who might be best supported in this way would be newly registered practitioners. It has been suggested that this function might be fulfilled by a preceptor who would be a role model and would help the novice nurse to develop day-to-day practice in the area in which they both work. The preceptor would be an experienced knowledgeable nurse who would be willing and able to prepare for this role.

Opportunities for development

Educational opportunities for professional development have increased considerably in recent years. It should be possible for most nurses to find some means of pursuing learning. There are of course the well established academic or professional courses, such as a degree in a nurse-related qualification such as psychology, sociology or biological sciences through a university or polytechnic; the diploma in nursing and ENB professional courses in critical care nursing; care of the elderly; and many other specialist nursing courses.

There has also been a rapid expansion in learning opportunities through open and distance learning. These enable the participant to learn at their own pace, in their own place. There are a range of institutions offering such learning packages. Most notable are the Open University, which is developing its nurse-related courses; the Distance Learning Centre for nursing at the South Bank Polytechnic and Barnet College, which offers a range of nurse-related packages, including the diploma in nursing which is validated by London University; and the English National Board which has also produced a series of learning packages for nurses. In addition, there are local initiatives for learning through courses, study days, workshops and conferences in topical subjects.

In fact for many nurses and their managers there are so many choices they have difficulty knowing what is best to do and finding the time and money to pursue their chosen path. Career advice becomes increasingly necessary with the growing provision and changing needs.

Retention of staff

It is said that regular training opportunities will keep nurses in nursing. It is estimated that about three quarters of nurses in employment would consider undertaking further education or training. Responsibility for meeting the learning needs and career development of nurses must be shared between management and employees.

Management needs to match individual skills and interests to both short and long term requirements of the organization. They also need to make sure that there are resources available to meet the needs, both human and financial. They should also provide support and mentorship to employees and be prepared to give feedback and rewards where they are merited.

Employees should show a commitment and interest in professional growth and should take the initiative in determining goals and matching these with the needs of the organization.

Part-time staff

It is vital that no employees are discriminated against in the pursuit of professional development, just because they work part-time or on a casual basis. Opportunities should be available equally to both part-time and full time staff. Problems faced by the casual employee are:

- Timing of learning opportunities which must take into consideration family commitments or other work.
- Venue where the learning takes place must be convenient for travel and parking.
- Repeat sessions should be arranged for people who are unavoidably ill or detained at work.
- What is offered must be well planned and relevant – organized to meet the objectives and needs of the participants and should be kept flexible.

There is no doubt that as nurses look to their future in nursing, whether they stay put or want to move upwards or sideways, they will have to engage in some form of continuing education or professional development. The big issues today are not will I or won't I but rather what shall I do? What is most appropriate? In making the choices it may help to have some idea of the way nursing is going as we approach the 21st century. The next chapter will give some indication of the possibilities.

References

Project 2000 Papers, United Kingdom Central Council (UKCC)
  First Report – A New Preparation for Practice (May 1986).
  Project Paper 1 – Introducing Project 2000 (Sept 1985).
  Project Paper 2 – The Learner: Student Status Revisited (Sept 1985).
  Project Paper 3 – One-Two-Three: How many levels of nurse should there be? (Sept 1985).

Project Paper 4 – The Enrolled Nurse: Looking back and looking forward (Sept 1985).
Project Paper 5 – Redrawing the Boundaries (Nov 1985).
Project Paper 6 – Facing the Future (Nov 1985).
Project Paper 7 – Results of the UKCC Consultation on Project 2000 (Jan 1987).
Project 2000 – Government Approval in Principle (May 1988).

DHSS (1988) *Which Way?* HMSO, London.
King's Fund Institute (1986) *Survey of continuing professional education.* King's Fund Institute, London.
Mavroleon, M. (1989) *The Second Time Around.* Unpublished project, Oxfordshire Health Authority.
Oxfordshire Regional Health Authority (1988) *Educational Strategy for Nursing.* Oxfordshire Regional Health Authority.
Poole, A. (1989) *Strategy for Nursing.* Department of Health, Nursing Division, London.
Report of the Committee on Nursing. Chairman Professor Asa Briggs, October 1972. HMSO, London.
South Bank Polytechnic Distance Learning Centre (1989) *Developing Professionally.* South Bank Polytechnic Distance Learning Centre.
United Kingdom Central Council (1984) *Code of Professional Conduct.* 2nd edn. UKCC, London.
United Kingdom Central Council (1990) *Post-registration Education and Practice Project (PREPP) – discussion paper.* UKCC, London.
United Kingdom Central Council (1990) Targets for health for all: Implications for Nursing/Midwifery (1986). *UKCC Register*, UKCC, London.
United Kingdom Central Council (1992) *Code of Professional Conduct.* 3rd edn. UKCC, London.

European Communities Directives
    77/452/EEC, 77/453/EEC and 77/454/EEC
    1977: *Official Journal of the European Communities*, 20(L 176).
    89/595/EEC
    1989: *Official Journal of the European Communities*, No. L 341/30.

Chapter 10
The Future

It is comparatively easy to look back, to reminisce, to recall life as it was many years ago. It is much more difficult to look forward with any clarity or certainty of life in general, or nursing in particular. Fifty or so years ago changes seemed to happen at a much slower, more acceptable rate, allowing people to assimilate one before they moved on to the next. Today change is occurring so rapidly on several fronts at the same time that it is nearly impossible to predict what the final outcome might be for any given change. For nurses returning after several years out of the profession it is hard enough trying to make sense of the changes that have taken place while they have been away, without looking forward to possible changes in the future.

Past predictions

In December 1969 Miss Priscilla Cooper gave her predictions for the future of nursing to the *Oxford Chronicle* on taking up an appointment as Chief Nursing Officer for Oxfordshire Health Authority.

On nurse preparation she said:

> 'We have to make sure we produce well trained nurses. I don't think we can go on with the present apprenticeship type training. In ten or five years even there will be no career outside the hospital service with an apprenticeship system. We have to realise young people now expect planned training and promotions. I hope there will be a real appreciation by the public of the need by everyone in the hospital services to give the nurses a very carefully planned education programme.'

On continuing education and retention of nurses:

> 'If we are to give patients really good care we have to preserve nurses for nursing and there must be a relief of long nursing duties. I think registered nurses will probably have to expand the various aspects of nursing. There could be a higher training and perhaps a

post registration course. Earlier in the century there was a limited choice of work for young women. It takes a lot more dedication for them to do nursing now, when there is such a choice of other careers with better pay and amenities.'

On links with medicine one of Miss Cooper's main views about medicine and nursing in the future is:

'the furtherance of the concept of total patient care with the closest possible links between the medical and nursing staff responsible for the preventive aspects of patient care. . . . we have to make sure nurses are properly used in the community and hospital and that there will be more links between the two.'

On enrolled nurses:

'I am a great believer in the two different types of training. There will be a demand for enrolled nurses who give wonderful patient care.'

On unqualified help:

'We have in many areas to enlist members of the community to help in the hospitals in the simplest ways. I am very keen on voluntary schemes which bring people in the community to help in hospitals. It is important that people should participate actively, especially where old people and children are concerned.'

Predictions fulfilled?

Miss Cooper did not make any suggestions as to how these predictions were to be achieved or in what time span. It is interesting 23 years later to determine how many of the predictions have been fulfilled.

As discussed in the previous chapter the changes in nurse preparation and the provision of continuing education for nurses after qualification have already been set in motion. The concept of total patient care has become central to the changes in the organization of nursing care, with the move away from task allocation to patient centred care.

However, forging close links between medicine and nursing and the preventive aspects of patient care have not been realized. Indeed it would appear that as nurses have, in some cases, quite radically changed the way they work, this has greatly disturbed doctors who see this as a threat to their control of patient care.

Links between hospitals and community services are not well developed. Community nursing has always appeared to be the 'poor relation' of hospital nursing, in the eyes of both the profession and the public. Some links have been made with the establishment of specialist nurses such as the parenteral nutrition sister or diabetic and paediatric liaison nurses, but these form only a small part of the total need of patients and nurses in the community.

Enrolled nurse

Although many people will agree with Miss Cooper's sentiments regarding the enrolled nurse, the profession as a whole felt that there was not a good enough case put forward for two levels of qualified nurse with different areas of responsibility. It was decided that one level of nurse would embrace most of the responsibilities of the two levels. This of course is in the process of being implemented but it is recognized that there could well be enrolled nurses working for another 40 years in jobs which will be protected.

Unqualified help

Miss Cooper's views on the use of unqualified helpers in hospital and encouraging voluntary schemes to bring people into hospitals to help, seem more altruistic than realistic in today's society. There is no doubt today of the need for the vast army of unqualified and mostly unpaid carers both in hospital and the community. The voluntary schemes tend to be support groups for patients suffering from specific conditions. They give advice and practical help to relatives and carers and raise funds to support research initiatives and to supply financial help where and when it is most needed. The League of Friends in hospitals and private nursing homes is another body of voluntary helpers who through fund raising efforts and refreshment stalls on the premises provide amenities and equipment for patients and staff which would not be available from other sources.

Miss Cooper concludes:

'I still think nursing is a very good career if you are truly interested in people.'

Is it possible to make predictions for the next 20 years with the same degree of accuracy as Miss Cooper? Only time will tell.

Goals of modern nursing

A major goal of modern nursing is to promote positive health.

'Health promotion is described as the process of enabling people to increase control over and improve their health, and to accept the community as the essential voice in matters of its own healthy living conditions and well-being.' From the Ottowa Charter drawn up by the World Health Organization in 1986.

This goal demands changes in attitudes and thinking by nurses in order to determine their targets for action.

In today's world, human needs are continually changing and similar action is required from the nursing profession if it is to respond to those needs. Such changes will be in the structure of society, with more frail elderly and young disabled people surviving and requiring support in their homes. People with life threatening conditions such as AIDS, and HIV positive sufferers, will need counselling and support in the community, as will those with other health problems related to contemporary lifestyles, such as alcohol and substance abusers, those with industrial diseases and those suffering from environmental pollution.

The traditional ideas of preserving life and promoting health are now enhanced by the recognition that individuals have responsibility for their own health and have the right to full information about the choices which face them. This requires the nurse to work in partnership with the patient or client in a wide variety of situations. It also requires greater flexibility on the part of the nurse to enable the specialist to work in both hospital and community settings.

New patterns of treatment and care will require changes in professional practice. Concepts of primary nursing, the nurse practitioner and the nurse consultant are now being tested and evaluated. Another role now emerging is that of lecturer/practitioner, which is attempting to bridge the theory practice gap. These developing roles aim to enable the practitioner to offer the highest level of care commensurate with their experience and qualifications.

Every major nursing setting should have links with a recognized centre of nursing research, both as a resource for information and a practice base for continuing research.

Tomorrow's nurse will need to use the computer with confidence, whether in a hospital or community setting. It will be the primary source of information and the primary method of recording data and instructions.

Project 2000 nurse

The new nurse preparation from Project 2000 should produce nurses with a different conception of nursing, able to analyse, problem solve and make decisions from a sound nursing knowledge base. These nurses should therefore be much more flexible and adaptable to changes as they occur. This will be necessary to cope with the rapid changes in technology in the acute sector of health care, and with the growing demands of the community sector. How nurses are deployed and the content and organization of nursing will become important in the recruitment and retention of nurses in the future.

Availability of manpower

The oft-quoted demographic time-bomb for the 1990s, in which there is a dramatic fall in the number of possible recruits for nursing because of a fall in the number of eighteen-year-olds leaving school, represents a major challenge to the future of nursing. At the same time the number of employment opportunities for women has increased considerably, particularly with the equal opportunities legislation which prevents employers from discriminating against women on the grounds of sex. This also means that women have raised expectations in terms of job satisfaction, career development and material rewards.

Role of management

The basis for any change in the future has to begin with management. The old idea of uncritical obedience, a rigid hierarchy and an undervaluing of nursing work is no longer appropriate. Nursing must be rewarding work for both men and women in order to retain them in the profession. The very human needs for esteem, recognition and self actualization are not satisfied where role expansion and professional responsibility are limited or denied.

It is the qualified nurses at the bedside who are in the best position to manage the care of the patient. They will of course need advice and support from other members of the health care team and a range of resources in order to function effectively.

It has been argued that within the NHS, nursing staff do not need to be managed by a nurse. There are some Health Authorities where the unit general manager has no nurse manager at a higher level than the senior nurse. A few nurses do have executive management positions but the vast majority prefer to remain in clinical contact with the patient. It is possible to achieve both job satisfaction and a support style of management if basic changes in practice and management are made.

Qualified nurses are already accountable for their professional practice. This is recognized in the Code of Professional Conduct published by the UKCC. They are primarily accountable to their patients to give quality care of a high standard. It is the patients who give the nurse the authority to act always in their best interests. These interests may be met through a system of primary nursing where an experienced qualified nurse determines care over a 24 hour period for the length of a patient's stay in hospital, or through a system of team nursing where an experienced qualified nurse leads a team of nurses to give care as before.

The responsibility for such a system is recognized in clinical grading where the nurses are usually paid on a sister grade or above. Although responsibility for management of patient care at delivery point will be with the primary nurse or team leader, there will still be a need for someone to co-ordinate and organize the nursing work at ward or departmental level.

Whatever this person is called – ward sister, senior nurse, co-ordinator or other name – the responsibilities will be similar , i.e., to act as clinical expert teaching and advising; leaders and disciplinarians within their field of activity; directors and organizers of nursing activities, liaising with other bodies as appropriate; and creators of and inspiration for the team as a whole to work together with mutual support in the best interests of the patients. These roles can apply equally to hospital or community settings.

Community work

It is estimated that more than 50% of nurses work outside the hospital setting, in community work of some kind. This work is diverse, covering the general population from birth to death including sickness prevention, screening services and support of chronically sick and disabled people in their own homes.

It came as a great disappointment therefore to nurses working in the community that their contribution was hardly recognized in the Griffiths II (1989) report. This report recommended that the bulk of responsibility for organizing and managing community services for everyone should be placed in the hands of the Social Services whom they believed were best placed to assess individual needs for services. Some see this as a cynical political move to shift responsibility for provision of care for an increasing number of elderly, sick and disabled people out of the NHS into local government through Social Services. There is a continuing debate on how all this is to be funded, locally or nationally.

Current position of community nurses

Nurses themselves must take part of the blame for the lack of recognition of the valuable work they do in the community. They have over the years fragmented their efforts and jealously guarded their professional boundaries. They have failed to move with the times and develop themselves professionally. A recent report (1991) from the PREPP department of the United Kingdom Central Council highlights these issues in the proposals it makes for the future of Community Education and Practice.

The proposals recognize the need for change to meet contemporary health care needs and to respond to changes in service provision and legislation. It is also felt that the duplication and fragmentation of post registration nursing education need to be addressed. Key features of the proposals suggest that a unified discipline of Community Health Care Nursing, with a shared common core, would offer greater choice and flexibility for the practitioner. A credit system would need to be established which recognized the value of previous experience and included opportunities for Enrolled Nurses.

Future community nursing roles

There is the potential for nurses to take key roles in the future in developing community nursing services to meet the demands of a discerning public, and at the same time to enhance the profile of nurses in the community. How this could be organized is difficult to determine but possibilities are:

- The nurse becoming an independent practitioner with her own clientele.
- The nurse functioning within a Health Centre or General Practice setting.
- Community nurses working in a particular locality, maybe even resident and acting as the local health advisors.

There have been some attempts in the past by nurses to try and establish themselves as independent clinical practitioners, but without any marked success. Reasons for this vary from resistance and down-right opposition from medical staff, who perhaps fear an erosion of their power and authority, to a lack of knowledge of both the effect and outcome of nursing practice.

As nurses become far more critical and less accepting of practice, as they question the reasons why and are prepared to take risks and introduce innovations in practice, so nursing can develop into a pro-fession which can offer a high level of service wherever and whenever it is needed.

Effective use of skills

Blanket statements – such as a philosophy which requires that all patients deserve to be cared for by a qualified nurse – can be restrictive and at times counter-productive. There are some aspects of care which can well be undertaken by experienced people who may not necessarily have a formal qualification. Nurses need to examine critically how they use their time and skills. They need to ask if they are making the most effective or efficient use of both, particularly as resources become more finite. Managers may well be asking these very questions soon, as they prepare budgets and monetary forecasts in future years.

In building up a team for a particular ward or department, a manager would be wise to take into consideration the total needs of the work area, and to put together a group of people who can fulfil different functions within the team. For instance, although newly qualified nurses can offer up-to-date knowledge, youth and enthusiasm, they will also need support and a possible role model as they move into a new area of practice. A mature nurse, perhaps returning to practice, is often seen as an asset even though possibly only able to offer part-time hours to start with. Such a person can give the team maturity, stability and life experience from which all team members and patients can benefit.

There is a need for leaders but there is also a need for workers, for innovators and maybe visionaries. These people may cross professional boundaries but in the process will enhance the care of the patient; one thing all professionals have in common is the need for good communication skills.

Working as a team

In developing care plans, nurses seek a contribution from all health care workers involved with the patient. Some do so verbally but more and more are prepared to share their assessment and plan in writing. As therapists move towards a degree-based training and consider common core subjects similar to nursing, dare we hope for more collaboration in preparation for professional qualification, with a shared degree in health care studies branching into specialist qualification in the final year? This can only improve mutual understanding and dissolve professional boundaries which can be detrimental to total patient care.

Support worker

Another piece to fit in the jig-saw puzzle of the future of nursing is the support worker. Nurses have a clear opportunity and responsibility in the future to get the support worker they would like. They are in the best position to decide the most appropriate work for unskilled help and to give the training needed to carry out that work to the highest possible standard. This is helped by the government initiative of awarding vocational qualifications for all employees who reach the required standard. Competencies to meet these standards have already been agreed by the professional bodies.

It is now the responsibility of the profession to accept the need not only to employ unqualified members in their teams but also to ensure that they have the opportunity and support in acquiring 'proper' training for the work they are expected to do as part of that team.

Societal influences

Nursing in the future cannot escape the broader effects of working patterns in the country. With an ageing workforce, a sharp increase in the number of married women working, and motherhood being only a temporary cessation of paid work, the demand for part-time work will increase. Fewer people will be committed to a life-time career working full time. There will be movement in and out of nursing with a demand for 'in-touch' facilities and professional up-dating.

With the move towards Health Authorities becoming purchasers and providers of health services, the likelihood of short fixed-term contracts for professional services will increase, especially as management is devolved down to smaller and smaller units, with loose links, contracting work from each other. For continuity and stability there will be a need for a small, core, full time workforce who will be supported by a larger, satellite, part-time workforce that can be more flexible.

For their support, part-time or contract employees will expect terms and conditions of work which will outweigh the disadvantages of part-time work. They will require hours to suit their lifestyle, and chances of promotion and career development and job satisfaction.

Whatever happens in the future, nursing is not and will never be a profession for those who seek an easy life. It is for those who want challenge, commitment and achievement. Nursing is togetherness, exploration, discovery and above all else will give a meaningful life to any who wholeheartedly embrace it.

Further reading

Books

Annual Report 1988–9 English National Board for Nursing, Midwifery & Health Visiting, London.

Bearshaw, V. & Robinson, R. (1990) *New for Old? Prospects for Nursing in the '90s.* McGraw-Hill Co. (UK) Ltd.

Davies, C. (1990) *Collapse of the Conventional Career.* Project Paper 1. English National Board for Nursing, Midwifery & Health Visiting, London.

DHSS Central Office of Information (1988) *Which Way?* HMSO, London.

Nursing in the '90s. Research Report 8. King Edward VII Hospital Fund for London, London.

Nursing Division (1989) *A Strategy for Nursing*. Department of Health Nursing Division, London.

Lysaught, J.P. (1981) *Action in Affirmation: Towards an Unambiguous Profession of Nursing*. McGraw-Hill Co. (UK) Ltd.

Oxfordshire Regional Health Authority (1988) *Education Nursing Strategy for Nursing*, Oxfordshire Regional Health Authority.

Ryan, D. (1990) *Project 1999 – The Support Hierarchy*, Department of Nursing Studies, University of Edinburgh.

Tatton, C. (1989) *2001 – The Black Hole – a Local Analysis*. Oxfordshire Health Authority.

Articles

Cooper, P. (1969) Nurses lead a normal life. *United Oxford Hospitals Chronicle*, December 1969, No. 8.

Cowling, C. (1990) Mandatory refreshment for nurses: an incentive to return. *Journal of Advanced Nursing*, **90**(15) 855–8.

Salvage, J. (1990) Nurses: the point of no return. *British Medical Journal*, 300 1478.

Index

Accountability, 49, 66, 68
Activities of living, 71
Adult learner, 49
Age, 99
Aide, 25
Application forms, 106
Approval for P.2000, 113
Apron, 57
Aromatherapy, 61
Assessment, 71, 101
Attitudes, 56, 87
Authority to act, 126
Availability, 44

Bank nursing, 100
Bed pan, 11
Beds, 61
Beliefs about nursing, 69
Boredom, 35
Bunsen burner, 12
Bureaucracy, 6
Business manager, 24

Care planning, 74
Carer, 21
CATS, 117
Changes, 49, 55
Childcare provision, 19, 40, 98
Child rearing, 19
Classroom, 87
Clinical placement, 84
Code of conduct, 66
Collar and cuffs, 57
Communications, 22
Community nursing, 127
Conditions of service, 96
Confidence, lack of, 17
Continuing education, 114
Contracts for supplies, 62
Cost, 46, 111

Course, 45
Culottes, 57

Day surgery, 64
Death, 14
Decision making, 69
Director of nursing, 3
Discipline, 4
Discontent, 96
Disincentives, 97
Disposal systems, 60
Distance learning, 46
Divorce, 35
Doing 'it', 47
Dressings, 60
Drugs, 37, 60, 82
Duvets, 61

Educational opportunities, 119
Enrolled nurses, 124
Environment, 59
Equipment, 11, 59, 60
Evaluation of care, 77
Expanding role, 66

Family responsibilities, 39
Fear, 37
Finance, 22
Fire drill, 82
Flexible hours, 98
Friendliness, 86

Generic nurse, 36
Goals personal, 101
Goal setting, 73
Grading, 96
Guidelines for re-entry, 44
Guilds, 9
Guilt, 36

Hats, 57
Health and safety, 81
Hierarchy, 6
Homemaker, 22
Home responsibilities, 39
Housework, 19

Implementation of care, 75
Incentives, 97
Incontinence sheets, 61
Infection control, 80
Informality, 56
Interpersonal skills, 25
Interview, 106

Job
    advertisements, 104
    application, 105
    security, 99
    status, 99

Knowledge, 66

Learning needs, 83
Leisure, 29
Letter writing, 106
Life experiences, 18

Management, 126
Matron, 34
Meals, 62
Medical advances, 64
Mentor, 84
Model of care, 70
Money, 33
Motivation, 41
Motivators, 41

Name badge, 59
National uniform, 58
Need for course, 47
Nightingale, 7
Nostalgia, 35
Nurse preparation, 109
Nursing process, 71
Nurturing, 19

Obedience, 5
Omission, 69
Organisation of care, 68, 95
Orientation, 86
Overseas, 28

Pace of change, 55
Partnership, 50, 57, 73
Part time staff, 120
Patient, 13, 57
Pay, 96, 102
Personal factors, 103
Plastic aprons, 58
Post reg. education, 113
Practice, 11
Preceptor, 119
Predictions, 122
Preparation for clinical placement, 79
PREPP, 114
Prevention of back injury, 82
Primary nursing, 76
Problem identification, 73
Professional practice, 66
Professional profile, 117
Programme framework, 112
Project 2000, 110, 125

Reality, 88
Reception, 86
Recruitment and retention, 119
Reminiscences, 1
Retraining, 43
Review system, 117
Rubbish, 60

Self assessment, 101
Services, 62
Sharps, 60
Single status, 34
Single level nurse, 111
Skill mix, 94
Socialisation, 9
Sources of information, 72
Specialised nursing, 64
Staffing shortages, 93
Standards for practice, 116
Statuary requirement, 43
Steriliser, 12
Studying, 27
Supernumary status, 111
Support, 57
Support worker, 112, 129
Systematic approach, 71

Tabards, 58
Task allocation, 75
Teams, 76, 129
Technology, 23, 38
Telephone call, 105

Theatre, 13
Theory, 10
Theory/practice gap, 95, 116
Training, 10
    environment, 112
    schools, 9
Travel, 98
Trousers, 57
Turnover – patient, 63

Unexpected, 86
Uniform, 57
Unsafe practice, 48

Vocation, 8
Voluntary work, 25

Ward sister, 95, 127
What work? 100, 103
Which course? 45